Midlife Metamorphosis

The Journey From Diet Culture to Radical
Acceptance

Mindy Gorman-Plutzer CHHC, CEPC, FNLP

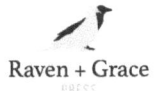

Raven + Grace
PRESS

Raven + Grace Press

Disclaimer

The information provided in this book is intended for educational purposes only and is not a substitute for professional medical advice, diagnosis, or treatment. Always seek the advice of your physician or other qualified health provider with any questions you may have regarding a medical condition. Neither the author nor the publisher assumes any liability for any loss, damage, or inconvenience resulting from the use or application of the information in this book.

Dedication

This book is dedicated to many:

To the hundreds of women who have allowed me to walk with them in their shoes,

To Jill, who's courage and strength taught me that desire can be bigger than fear,

To Ricki and Dani as we continue to honor the past, celebrate the present, and embrace all that is yet to come.

And to Eddie, for believing in me when I wasn't able to

Contents

Before We Begin

Since writing my first book, *The Freedom Promise*, in 2013, I've exponentially evolved in both my professional practice and personal journey. With my certification in functional medicine nutrition counseling, I've been able to bring a fresh perspective to the remarkable women who come to me struggling with their relationship with food and their bodies. These women—bright, insightful, and courageous—often experience digestive discomfort, hormonal fluctuations, mood changes, and anxiety, either contributing to or resulting from their food challenges.

Every day, I have the privilege of working with the most extraordinary women, open-hearted, receptive, and deeply committed to their inner journey. They dive courageously into the heart of their stories with me, creating a space of trust where transformation becomes not just possible but inevitable. This connection and the possibility of your own beautiful transformation are my greatest hopes for these pages.

This Book Is for You If:

You can no longer bear the weight of deprivation.

You're overwhelmed by conflicting nutritional information.

You're navigating midlife changes and find yourself turning to food for comfort.

You're ready to stop blaming your "willpower" and instead empower yourself to stop dieting and start living.

You're in recovery and would benefit from compassionate support.

Do your food choices reflect what you believe you've "earned" rather than what truly nourishes you? Do you approach social gatherings with anxiety about "losing control"? Do you wake with thoughts immediately focused on weight and body size? Are you using food to self-medicate? Do you believe you've "tried everything" yet still struggle with food thoughts, behaviors, and weight?

YOU ARE NOT ALONE. You stand among millions of women navigating their relationship with food. I understand that you may also experience digestive challenges, mood fluctuations, and anxiety.

You are not broken. You haven't failed. The methods you've relied on are failing you. You know how to diet but may be confused about how to truly nourish yourself. Overeating or under-eating are messengers pointing toward something deeper calling for your attention.

What This Book Is (And Isn't): A Midlife Perspective

This book isn't another diet program; though if you follow these steps and adopt these strategies, your body will likely find its happy, healthy weight as you release food's hold on you. It's definitely not designed to diagnose or cure psychological issues contributing to your relationship with food.

What it IS designed for is helping you reclaim power taken by a $163.13 billion diet industry[1] intent on filling you with falsehoods and myths that undermine your capacity to trust what truly nourishes you. The industry has targeted you for decades, profiting from your dissatisfaction with your body, and has convinced you that aging is a problem to be solved rather than a privilege to be embraced.

You will navigate confusion surrounding nutrition, so you can finally stop fearing what food will do TO you and embrace the nourishing wisdom of what food can do FOR you. I'll introduce you to the physiology at the root of your symptoms and help you discover how it impacts the psychology driving your behaviors. Conversely, I'll explore the psychology behind your behaviors and how it affects your physiology.

---

1. Market Research Future (MRFR), *"Weight Loss and Weight Management Diet Market Research Report,"* 2024.

You'll learn that HOW, WHY, and WHEN we eat profoundly impacts WHAT we eat. I'll guide you toward making empowered choices from within–from a place of gratitude, acceptance, and forgiveness. You'll discover how to honor your appetite (for appetite is life) and how stress sabotages your efforts toward the body you desire. You'll find relief knowing that punishing exercise isn't necessary and discover movement that honors your body rather than attempting to make it disappear. For women in midlife, this reframing of movement becomes especially liberating. Your body deserves gentle care and joyful movement, not punishment for existing in its natural state.

You'll come to understand that food and nourishment are more than calories, developing respect for their colorful, intricate beauty. You'll learn practices connecting you to your body's wisdom, helping you discern which foods serve your unique needs. I'll share my nearly half-century experience with limiting beliefs and destructive food behaviors. I'll offer my philosophy, often supported by relevant science, for living the big, beautiful, truly nourished life I enjoy today. Plus, you'll receive actionable steps toward experiencing the FREEDOM you deserve, plus additional resources from respected leaders in the field.

I share stories from women, like you, who grew weary of feeling deprived and depleted. Please note that all names have been changed to protect their privacy. And finally, I'll invite you to explore nourishment beyond food entirely, as you discover the gifts that come with radical and compassionate acceptance.

What Is Radical Acceptance?

Radical acceptance is the profound practice of embracing reality exactly as it is, without resistance, judgment, or attempts to force change. At its core, it means completely accepting your present situation, thoughts, feelings, and experiences–particularly the painful or difficult ones–without trying to change them, fight against them, or judge them as good or bad. It's about acknowledging "what is" rather than focusing on "what should be."

The key elements include: acknowledging reality exactly as it is, even when it's painful; recognizing that suffering comes not just from pain itself but from resistance to pain; letting go of the struggle against reality; understanding that acceptance doesn't mean approval or giving up; and practicing mindful awareness of thoughts and feelings without judgment.

Radical acceptance doesn't mean resignation or passivity. Rather, it creates a foundation of clarity from which effective action can emerge. By fully accepting your current reality, you gain the emotional freedom and mental clarity to make conscious choices about how to respond to situations rather than reacting from a place of fear, denial, or resistance.

My hope is that you'll emerge enlightened, inspired, and motivated to transform your relationship with food and your body–from one rooted in fear and confusion to a relationship offering authentic nourishment. If how we approach one aspect of life reflects how we approach everything, this newly nourished version of yourself can only emerge as brilliant and magnificent.

I want you to experience how being truly nourished creates an expanded presence rather than the diminished one that emerges when we exhaust our energy trying to become smaller.

Let's get started.

Introduction

The Path to Radical Acceptance

"In the infinity of life where I am, all is perfect, whole, and complete. I now choose to calmly and objectively see my old patterns, and I am willing to make changes. I am teachable. I can learn. I am willing to change. I choose to have fun while doing this. I choose to react as though I have found a treasure when discovering something else to release. I see and feel myself changing moment by moment. Thoughts no longer have any power over me. I am the power in my world. I choose to be free. All is well in my world." – Louise Hay

The Roots of My Story: Where It All Began

I was eight years old, setting the table for my baby sister Jill's second birthday, when I innocently remarked to my father how quickly she'd grow up. His face turned ashen, his eyes squinting with that familiar anger, and I wanted to crawl under the table, bewildered by what I'd said wrong. Soon after, I learned the devastating truth. Jill had been diagnosed with cystic fibrosis, with a life expectancy of just two years. A heavy, foreboding cloud descended over our home as we concealed her condition to protect my parents' fear of being stigmatized, while I laid in bed night after night listening to her frightful cough, praying she wouldn't die.

In this crisis, I learned that it was incumbent upon me to cause no trouble, stay out of the way, help with household chores, and align my behavior and opinions with what my parents valued. I became the ultimate people-pleaser, never developing a strong sense of self. For me, love became control and respect became obedience, as I desperately sought approval and connection from parents who struggled to connect themselves. The foundation was set for a lifetime of seeking external validation over internal truth.

Without a strong connection to myself and defining my successes by things outside of myself, I never felt safe. Restricting my food and pushing my body to be smaller became the only way I could feel in control. Was I seeking attention? Did I want to disappear? Was my feeling of not being enough driving me to never be satisfied that I was thin enough? Probably yes, yes, yes.

My expertise comes not only from textbooks, but from lived experience. I understand the intricate web of food restriction, body hatred, and emotional numbing because I've been trapped in it. I know what it feels like to step on the scale multiple times a day, to calculate calories obsessively while appearing to live a "perfect" life, to panic over dinner invitations, and to measure self-worth by the size of your body.

My relationship with dieting and yearning for a different body began in my teens. Always thin as a child, I began to naturally round out during puberty. Restricting calories was a way of life in our home, and as the obedient daughter, I embraced this practice with determination. I absorbed the belief that "bad" foods made you fat, and fat was undesirable, as well as unacceptable.

Through the years, I witnessed and participated in countless diet trends. The scale became the voice that answered my daily question: "Am I good enough?" I measured my worth by the size of my body, but my perception was distorted. I had lost the ability to see myself clearly, to connect with the wisdom of my body.

The College Years and Beginning of Family Life

College in the 1970s introduced new methods of controlling my appetite such as amphetamines prescribed for all-night studying and the recreational substances that were supposedly non-addictive. Some days consisted solely of Tab (the popular diet soft drink) and Light n' Lively Ice Milk. I discovered alcohol and late-night munchies, sending my weight on wild fluctuations.

During my final year of college, I met Stuart, who would soon become my husband. Not too long after we married I was pregnant with our first daughter. Determined not to carry extra baby weight, I obsessively counted calories, managing to gain just twenty pounds. Fifteen months later, pregnant again and increasingly disconnected from my body's wisdom, I proudly kept my weight gain to only seventeen pounds while delivering another healthy daughter weighing over seven pounds.

By my mid-thirties, being the thinnest person in the room had become my obsession. I stepped on the scale countless times daily. We were blessed with a beautiful life–the country club membership, community involvement, and wonderful friendships. Yet something essential was missing. Me. I struggled to find peace in my own skin.

I would panic over dinner plans while secretly eating beforehand, meticulously measure wine at home but order multiple glasses when dining out. Balancing a household budget challenged me, yet I could calculate the precise calorie count of any meal without hesitation. It was, quite simply, insanity.

Eventually, I recognized my need for help. My schedule was filled with weekly weigh-ins, meal plans, and therapy sessions. Despite my struggles, I possessed the wisdom not to subject my daughters to the diet nightmares I had experienced. We all needed healing, and deep within, I knew this work centered on self-acceptance and releasing the pressure to become what I perceived to be a "better" version of myself.

Navigating Loss and Finding Purpose

In 1995, I began working at a nutritional counseling center, sharing weight loss secrets that had held me captive for years. The irony wasn't lost on me; I was being paid to perpetuate the very system that had caused me so much suffering. For seven years, I guided clients through the same restrictive patterns I was still struggling to break free from myself. This experience taught me invaluable lessons about the limitations of traditional approaches to food and weight.

What makes me uniquely qualified to guide you isn't just my personal recovery; it's the depth of my understanding of both sides of this struggle. I've been the client desperate for answers and the professional trying to provide them within a broken system. I've witnessed firsthand how traditional diet culture fails women repeatedly, and I've spent decades studying what actually works.

I continued my education in nutrition and psychology, but my real expertise comes from understanding that this journey isn't about willpower or finding the "right" diet. It's about healing your relationship with yourself. I've learned that sustainable change happens not through restriction and control, but through radical acceptance and self-compassion.

Life appeared perfect in my mid-forties when Stuart was diagnosed with stage four metastatic melanoma. After a long battle lasting twenty-one months, we lost him in August 2004. Grief unfolded in complex layers. At forty-nine years old, I faced single motherhood, financial responsibility, and the search for a new purpose. I turned to alcohol—not social drinking, but desperate numbing. I recognized this as an extension of my disordered eating patterns.

This period taught me that healing isn't linear and that true recovery means learning to navigate life's inevitable challenges without returning to destructive coping mechanisms.

My Sister's Journey and A Personal Revelation

During these years of personal struggle and healing, my sister Jill continued her remarkable journey with cystic fibrosis. While her condition presented enormous challenges, she lived with extraordinary grace and resilience. We lost Jill in 2014, she was fifty-three years old, and at that time, a rarity among cystic fibrosis patients. She had lived a life that defied all medical expectations, full of love, purpose, and meaning despite the daily challenges of her condition.

As I moved forward, honoring her memory, I began experiencing symptoms that led to my own diagnosis of atypical cystic fibrosis in 2023. After decades of battling my body, I finally made peace with it, only to face this unexpected health challenge.

This diagnosis has become another layer of my expertise. I now understand intimately what it means to practice radical acceptance when facing a chronic health condition. I know how to maintain a loving relationship with your body even when it doesn't behave as you'd hoped. I've learned to care for my health from a place of compassion rather than control, which is precisely what I teach my clients about their relationship with food.

Life Today: Embracing the Fullness of Being

As I enter my seventh decade, I find myself in a place of profound gratitude and joy that once seemed unimaginable. I am happily remarried to a wonderful man who not only supports my growth but actively encourages me to stand in my value every single day. Together, we've created a rich and meaningful life surrounded by our children and eight extraordinary grandchildren. In fact, becoming a grandmother was a powerful catalyst that inspired me to fully embrace what had been brewing in the early years of seeking recovery and food freedom.

There is something about looking into the eyes of a grandchild that crystallizes what truly matters. Their pure, unconditional love helped me realize that I wanted to be fully present, not just physically, but emotionally and spiritually, for every moment we share. This meant finally releasing the last vestiges of food preoccupation and body dissatisfaction that had shadowed parts of my life for so long.

My diagnosis came during this time of authentically standing in my value, yet it has called upon me to practice radical, yet compassionate acceptance at an entirely new level. Each day now, as I care for my health with necessary treatments and medications, I do so from a place of love and respect for my body rather than resentment or despair.

In truth, my life has never been richer or more meaningful than it is today. My professional work with women seeking their own food freedom brings profound fulfillment. After decades of personal struggle and professional experience, I understand that lasting transformation requires addressing the whole person—not just eating behaviors, but the underlying beliefs, traumas, and patterns that drive them. I know that true freedom comes not from following another set of rules, but from learning to trust yourself again.

My expertise comes not only from textbooks, but from lived experience. I maintain my recovery while navigating real-life challenges: managing a chronic health condition, being a mother and grandmother who wants to model body acceptance, running a business, and maintaining meaningful relationships. This isn't theoretical knowledge; it's practical wisdom gained through decades of both struggle and triumph. I understand the intricate web of food restriction, body hatred, and emotional numbing because I've been trapped in it. More importantly, I know the path out.

The Gradual Clearing

You might wonder what exactly changed for me and when everything finally aligned. While some individuals can pinpoint the exact date of their last binge or drink, my recovery from disordered eating resembled a gradual clearing of the fog. As I educated myself about true nourishment, I slowly returned home to my body's wisdom.

I discovered joy in movement, moving my body with love rather than punishment. I explored my relationship with fear-based living and embraced the practice of integrity to self. None of this would have resonated without the extraordinary support of friends and professionals who continue to guide and champion me.

Freedom arrived in quiet moments of forgetting. One morning, I realized I hadn't thought about the scale in days. I walked out the door noticing how confident I felt rather than scrutinizing how my body looked. Restaurant invitations transformed from sources of dread into opportunities for connection and joy. Perhaps most powerful of all, I began filling candy bowls, their presence no longer a threat nor trigger. Liberation wasn't dramatic, but it was found in these small, everyday moments when food and body worries had simply faded into the background of a rich, full life.

I allowed myself to experience uncomfortable emotions and situations. I learned that no feeling is more uncomfortable than the discomfort of avoiding it. I allowed myself to appear vulnerable. I began having difficult conversations and discovered their liberating power. I acknowledged my insecurities and fears for what they were, which is False Evidence Appearing Real. I released the exhausting pursuit of perfection.

I began to understand what it truly means to be connected to my body, to feel present and alive. Being connected allows me to honor my hunger and satisfy what I'm genuinely longing for. I fell in love again, this time with myself. I discovered I am delightful company.

As my perspective transformed, I embraced that calories represent energy and that my body needs protein, fat, and carbohydrates to thrive. I can make empowered choices about the nutrients I offer my body, and yes, I can enjoy quality food while maintaining vibrant health. I trust myself with food, appreciating its complexity. Hunger is no longer a source of anxiety.

I eat what nourishes me when my body signals hunger, trusting that I'll recognize when I am satisfied. I engage in movement that brings joy and will honor my need for rest. I surround myself with people, places, and experiences that illuminate my purpose and fulfill my spirit. I've released relationships and situations that no longer serve my highest good.

Radical acceptance has served me well as I look back on a life filled with loss and disappointment. It has created, within me, a sacred and loving place to always return home to, my deepest self. This acceptance meant acknowledging my relationship with food, my body, and my grief as they truly existed, not as I wished them to be.

When I compassionately accepted my reality, I freed myself from the emotional energy previously consumed by resistance, shame, and judgment. This energy became available for genuine healing and growth. Today, I stand as living proof that no matter how long you've struggled, no matter how hopeless it may seem, transformation is possible when you embrace that it's less about what you do and more about what you accept and let go of in order to become the change. The change you want to see, experience and put out into the world.

Sitting here writing the introduction to my second book reminds me how far I've traveled. Imagine how far your journey might take you. Your time is now. It's time to stop trading the richness of your life for the size of your body.

With love and compassion,
Mindy

Chapter Summary

In this introduction, I share my deeply personal journey from a childhood marked by family dynamics that shaped my relationship with food, through decades of disordered eating patterns, to a place of radical acceptance and food freedom in my seventh decade of life. I reveal how family circumstances, including my sister Jill's cystic fibrosis diagnosis, influenced my early need to be perfect and please others, which later manifested in my very complicated relationship with food and body image.

Through navigating marriage, motherhood, widowhood, re-marriage, and my own health challenges with atypical cystic fibrosis, I hope my story illustrates how radical acceptance, embracing reality exactly as it is without resistance or judgment, became the foundation for my healing. The journey from food fear to food freedom offers hope for women in midlife who are ready to stop trading the richness of their lives for the size of their bodies.

Personal Reflection Exercises

Exercise 1: Recognizing Your Story's Origins

Take a few moments to reflect on your earliest memories related to food, eating patterns, and body awareness. Write freely for 10-15 minutes, allowing memories and insights to emerge without judgment. Consider these questions:

- What messages did you receive about food and body size in your childhood home?

- Were there family circumstances that may have influenced your relationship with food?

- When did you first become aware of your body size in relation to others?

- How were food and meals handled in your family? Were they sources of comfort, control, celebration, or anxiety?

Exercise 2 : The Messages We Carry

Create two columns on a page:

Column 1: External Messages

List the messages you've received about food, eating, and your body size from external sources (family, media, doctors, friends, diet culture, etc.). Be specific about what these messages told you about your worth, acceptability, and how you "should" be.

Column 2: My Inner Truth

Next to each external message, write what your inner wisdom knows to be true. What does the wisest part of you believe about your worthiness, your body's intelligence, and what nourishment truly means?

Exercise 3: Defining Radical Acceptance for Yourself

I describe radical acceptance as "the profound practice of embracing reality exactly as it is, without resistance, judgment, or attempts to force change."

Reflect on what radical acceptance means to you personally:

- What aspects of your relationship with food or your body do you find hardest to accept?

- How might your life be different if you could fully accept these aspects without judgment?

- What would you gain by releasing resistance to "what is" in your current reality?

- In what ways might acceptance create space for positive change rather than resignation?

- Write a personal definition of what radical acceptance means to you and how it might transform your relationship with food and your body.

Laying the Foundation, Re-framing the Story, Embracing Lasting Freedom

The Beauty of Starting Where You Are

"No book is just one chapter, no chapter tells the whole story, no mistakes define who we are. Keep turning the pages that are left to be turned." - Shannon L. Alder

For those who don't yet know me, my path to this work wasn't linear. At forty-nine, I found myself starting over in ways that felt vastly different than similar transitions in my thirties. The uncertainty and vulnerability were, at times, overwhelming. Now I see that midlife offered me exactly what I needed: the perfect combination of earned wisdom and remaining years to apply it meaningfully.

Through that experience—through navigating the landscape of fear with courage—I developed a strategy that has proven both repeatable and transformational. And here's the truth I discovered: There is no "wrong time" to begin. The richness you bring to this work now, your life experience, your deepened understanding of yourself, your capacity for self-reflection, these are not disadvantages. They are your greatest strengths.

You see, my fear and profound sense of inadequacy once manifested in how I treated my body. I couldn't be small enough. I hid behind a body that constantly fluctuated in size, my relationship with myself reflected my relationship with everything and everyone else. What I eventually discovered in my fifties was eye opening: My disordered eating wasn't the problem. It had become my solution, a misguided attempt to navigate a world where I feared I had no control.

This midlife revelation changed everything.

The breakthrough came when I realized my strategy could be taught, shared, and implemented across many life situations. Today, I've used these principles to create both subtle shifts and transformative changes–not just in my life, but in the lives of countless women I've had the honor to coach.

Most profoundly, I now connect with women in ways more meaningful than I ever dreamed possible.

The Gift of Midlife Transformation

As women reach midlife, we bring a clarity that only comes with time, a capacity to discern what truly matters, to recognize patterns more quickly, and to value our peace more than we value external validation. These are not small advantages.

There is something remarkably powerful about the transformation that occurs in our middle years. The masks we once wore become heavy. The performances grow tiresome. There emerges a beautiful readiness to simply be and to claim our truth without apology.

This approach to achieving sustainable results will help you be present in your body and experience food and movement in ways not overshadowed by concerns over size, shape, and numbers. You'll learn to navigate emotions and life experiences using strategies that don't compromise your health or well-being but, rather, enrich it by empowering you to embrace a healing relationship with food, one designed for genuine nourishment rather than mere weight restoration or loss.

This approach allows you to model for others how to eat a variety of foods in various settings and move for joy rather than compulsion. In this space, your relationship with your body becomes one of authentic self-acceptance, compassion, and forgive-ness. What a profound gift to offer younger generations by show-ing them a different way to inhabit their bodies than the punishing relationship you may have experienced.

You'll discover that your experiences aren't sim-ply part of being flawed. Rather, your iden-tity and relationship with food and body are complex, intertwined with your unique biology. Your challenges represent real emotions, fears, and insecurities that need acknowledgment and space. Healing is about creating that safe con-tainer while developing new practices of relat-ing to food, body, and self.

Truth in Nutrition at Midlife and Beyond

These are strange times for nutritionists. Conflicting trends like anti-diet movements and body positivity clash with obsessions over bio-hacking every minor ailment. The mantra "test, don't guess" has reached excessive levels, prompting people to scrutinize aspects that may not call for such attention or financial investment. (This is a term used by functional practitioners as we navigate making diagnosis or prescribing supplements, but it has gone too far with testing being expensive and marketable). The challenge lies in proper interpretation, in contextualizing results appropriately.

For women in midlife, this confusion is often compounded by changing nutritional needs, hormonal fluctuations, and decades of conflicting advice. Your body at forty-five, fifty-five, or sixty-five is not the same as it was at twenty-five and this is a natural evolution, not a flaw to be fixed. My role as a functional medicine nutritionist transcends mere prescriptions, diet plans, or rigid protocols. Keto, paleo, intermittent fasting, macrobiotic, plant-based...nutrition's complexity defies such simplification, especially in bodies with decades of lived experience.

In truth, simplified approaches often don't work, at least not sustainably, and certainly don't work without addressing deeper foundational elements.

Central to this foundation is understanding the CONTEXT into which nutrition fits such as the context of your unique body, the context within which YOUR relationship with food evolved. My concern extends beyond what you eat or your test results; it encompasses YOU, your journey, habits, and lived experience.

Your entirety–from birthplace and ancestral roots to adolescent experiences, current discomforts, sleep patterns, and daily rhythms–paints a far richer picture for true functional nutrition in practice than dietary choices or isolated test results ever could.

The Wisdom of Non-Negotiables: Ancient Wisdom for Modern Midlife

I often remind clients about the wisdom embedded in ancestral healing practices. While modern medicine has made remarkable advancements, we benefit tremendously from acknowledging that age-old traditions often contain valuable insights that complement medical interventions. These ancestral approaches emphasize the interconnectedness of mind, body, and spirit, alongside natural remedies and lifestyle adjustments.

For women in midlife, this ancient wisdom offers particular relevance. As our bodies shift and change, these fundamental principles provide stability and nourishment that trendy diets cannot match.

Throughout most of conventional medicine's history, core elements known as the "non-negotiables" were central to health management. First articulated over six thousand years ago in Ancient Greece, these included:

- Diet

- Sleep

- Exercise

- Breath

- Excretion

- Emotions

Beyond Greco-Roman traditions, several non-Western healing systems focus on food, digestion, and elimination as key aspects of healthy minds and bodies. Ayurvedic traditions in India base ideas of health around balancing the body through consuming foods with appropriate properties. Modern traditional Chinese medicine practices pay careful attention to systems for extracting energy from food and processing toxins. Traditional African and Native American medicines incorporate herbs focused on digestive health.

Despite our profound historical and cross-cultural connections to gut health and these core lifestyle factors, modern conventional medicine often overlooks their significance, creating a critical gap in our approach to wellness, particularly for women navigating midlife transitions.

This is where functional nutrition counselors shine. By leveraging ancient wisdom regarding vital connections between diet, digestion, and overall well-being, we bridge the gap between traditional knowledge and modern healthcare. Our role isn't to replace established medical procedures but to complement them. By integrating insights from both ancient wisdom and contemporary evidence, we offer a holistic approach to health that honors your body's changing needs.

We guide our clients towards addressing the underlying causes of their health issues. We educate about missing pieces in their health journey to support healing. We empower them to make a difference at home, decreasing dependency on medical teams while becoming better partners for their providers. We keep in mind that our clients are the experts of their experiences and hold the potential to become masters of their own healing. This is not to infer that you don't seek medical attention when needed or that you ignore evidence-backed recommendations. My message is to never forget that no one knows your body better than you do and it is your responsibility to speak up when you feel you are not being heard. If a doctor or practitioner isn't helping you to feel seen, find a new one.

And crucially, we're not just addressing symptoms. We're examining why those symptoms emerged in the first place. When we turn our attention to "what's happening within," "backing it up," and "connecting the dots", we consider gut health and digestion as primary roots of any chronic health challenge.

Honoring Your Journey, Embracing Your Future

Throughout this book, I won't guide you to change. Instead, I'll prompt you to release thoughts, beliefs, behaviors, and foods that no longer serve a useful purpose. I'll encourage you to explore not only WHAT you're eating but also WHO you are as an eater. I'll invite you to reframe your story in ways that honor 'what was' while creating new chapters that speak to your authentic self-expression. The potential is a happily ever after.

At midlife, this reframing takes on special significance. You have the opportunity to look at your story with compassionate eyes and to rec-

ognize how you've done the best you could with the tools you had available. This perspective is powerful; it allows you to see where you've been and where you're going.

I am deeply honored to walk this path with you.

Chapter Summary

In this foundational chapter, I introduced the unique gifts and opportunities that midlife offers for transformation. I explained how our relationship with food and body is not simply about willpower but about deeper patterns of relating to ourselves.

The chapter explores the shift from willpower to willingness, the power of gratitude to move us from scarcity to abundance, and the courage to face our feelings rather than numbing them with food. I introduced the concept that true nourishment extends beyond food to include relationships, purpose, and spirituality. By choosing love over fear and releasing limiting beliefs, we begin creating the foundation for lasting food freedom.

Personal Reflection Exercises

Exercise 1: Recognizing Your Story's Origins

Take a moment to reflect on the unique wisdom and clarity that has come with your years of life experience:

- What do you value now that perhaps didn't seem as important in your younger years?

- What concerns or worries have diminished with time and perspective?

- How has your definition of "success" or "happiness" evolved since your twenties or thirties?

- What strengths do you possess now that you didn't have earlier in life?

Write a letter to your younger self about the wisdom you've gained that you wish you had known then, particularly around food, body, and self-worth.

Exercise 2: Your Non-Negotiables Inventory

Reflect on the non-negotiables from ancient wisdom traditions (diet, sleep, exercise, breath, excretion, and emotions):

1. For each area, rate your current level of attention and care

on a scale of 1-10:

- Diet/Nourishment: _____

- Sleep quality and quantity: _____

- Movement/Exercise: _____

- Breath/Breathing awareness: _____

- Digestion/Elimination: _____

- Emotional awareness and regulation: _____

2. Choose one area that received a lower score. What is one small, sustainable change you could make in this area this week?

3. How might improving this foundational element affect your relationship with food?

Journal Prompts

1. **Scarcity vs. Abundance:** In what ways does a scarcity mindset show up in your relationship with food? What thoughts, beliefs, or behaviors reflect this perspective? How might you begin to shift toward an abundance mindset around nourishment?

2. **Midlife Evolution:** You've read that in midlife, "The

masks we once wore become heavy. The performances grow tiresome." What masks or performances around food, eating, or your body are you ready to release?

3. **Beyond Food Nourishment:** Reflect on the statement that "we're nourished by so much more than the food on our plates." What forms of non-food nourishment feel most fulfilling to you? Where might you be experiencing a nourishment deficit that food can't actually satisfy?

4. **Letting Go:** What thoughts, beliefs, or behaviors around food and body no longer serve you? What would become possible in your life if you could release them?

Eating Disorders in Midlife

Comprehending the Path to Complete Acceptance

While *Midlife Metamorphosis* isn't exclusively about eating disorder recovery, I feel called to honor how common these struggles are among women navigating midlife transitions. My own recovery journey is woven throughout these pages because it shaped how I understand the complex relationship we have with our bodies and food during this life stage.

I recognize that not every reader will share this particular struggle, and that's perfectly okay. For those who do find themselves in the grip of disordered eating patterns, whether recognized or hidden, I hope my vulnerability offers a beacon of possibility and hope. Recovery is real, and it's never too late to rewrite your story with food and your body.

For those whose journeys look different, my hope is that witnessing one woman's path to freedom might illuminate your own unique relationship with nourishment, self-acceptance, and the profound transformation that midlife can offer us all.

Young women going through adolescence and early adulthood are not the only individuals affected by eating disorders, contrary to popular belief. The truth is far more complex, as eating challenges in midlife are becoming more common in our culture. Only a small percentage of people who are struggling ever seek formal treatment, yet treatment centers nationwide report an increase in the number of women and men over thirty-five seeking help for these complex conditions. These statistics probably only represent the outward manifestation of a much larger problem that affects countless lives.

Naturally, one might speculate why these challenges are so prevalent in midlife. Understanding the particular changes and demands that this stage of life brings is the key to the solution. Significant marital disruptions, divorce, and mourning frequently leave emotional voids that seem impassable. Food behaviors may arise as an attempt to numb emotional pain or restore control in the midst of upheaval, as these losses can cause profound sorrow and uncertainty. The strain of providing care, whether for elderly parents, children, or both at once, also puts a great deal of strain on women in their middle years. While helping others, this "sandwich generation" frequently disregards their needs, which fosters the growth of disordered eating practices as improvised coping strategies.

Another important trigger, especially for women going through perimenopause and menopause, is hormonal shifts. Physiological changes resulting from these natural transitions affect mood regulation, metabolism, and body composition. Many women suffer from severe body image distress when these changes take place in a culture that values youthful bodies, and some women resort to disordered habits like dietary restriction in an effort to "control" their changing appearance. One's sense of self and purpose is also called into question during the empty nest time. When children move out, parents frequently find it difficult to realign their lives after decades of being primarily responsible for providing care. As they look for new sources of structure and purpose, this identity disruption may show itself as complex interactions with food.

The extremely negative messages about aging bodies in our Western culture are perhaps one of the most widespread triggers. More than eighty-eight percent of middle-aged women, according to research, express substantial body dissatisfaction. This study found that this large number of women aged fifty and older reported body dissatisfaction, with weight being a significant concern across this demographic. The research was part of the Gender and Body Image (GABI) study which specifically examined body image issues in this demographic of women.[1] Deep distress is caused by worries about weight redistribution, skin changes, and

---

1. Gagne, D. A., Von Holle, A., Brownley, K. A., Runfola, C. D., Hofmeier, S., Branch, K. E., & Bulik, C. M. (2012).

other normal aging processes. These natural changes can feel more like personal failures than normal parts of human development in a culture that values youth and beauty. As people try to stop or reverse the aging process by food manipulation, this unhappiness quickly turns into disordered eating. This image can be further complicated by financial strains and retirement transitions, which frequently lead to anxiety and identity loss, especially when careers have been essential to one's sense of self-worth and social connections.

In light of these potent triggers, what is the path to recovery and sustainable wellness? The solution is radical and compassionate acceptance, a life-changing strategy that can radically change how you relate to food and your body. Fundamentally, this concept entails accepting your current situation completely, without bias or opposition. This gives you the opportunity to observe things properly before choosing how to react, not to condone unpleasant situations or accept misery. This method is especially effective for healing from midlife eating disorders because it directly addresses the reluctance many people feel toward normal life transitions.

Recognizing your body's normal changes throughout life is the first step toward radical, yet compassionate acceptance. Recovery means embracing your body's knowledge and its right to change, rather than resisting unavoidable changes in look and function. To achieve this, the cultural narrative that physical alteration equates to moral failure or a lack of discipline must be contested. And who better to do this than our generation of women, as we are ever evolving. Similar to this, radical acceptance encourages embracing your whole spectrum of emotions rather than using food to numb bad feelings. You can acknowledge all feelings, especially the difficult ones, as natural components of your human experience rather than as dangers that need to be controlled by eating habits.

Releasing the perfectionism that frequently feeds midlife eating challenges is another step in the healing process. Many people exhaust themselves trying to achieve an unachievable ideal by adhering to strict guidelines and unrealistic standards for diet, exercise, and beauty. Realizing that you were never intended to stay the same despite life's changes requires that compassionate acceptance, which entails letting go of your perfectionism and creating space for self-compassion. Reconnecting with your body's natural understanding regarding hunger, fullness, and sustenance is facilitated by radical acceptance as you progress through your recovery. This entails having faith that your body will recognize what it needs when it is not restricted by cultural norms around "appropriate" eating or arbitrary dietary laws.

The most basic aspect of the journey from diet culture to food freedom and radical acceptance may be realizing that your worth has never been determined by how you look or how well you conform to social norms. In midlife, healing and sustainable wellness is finding your way back to more profound sources of meaning and purpose, whether via community service, artistic endeavors, spiritual pursuits, relationships, or other activities that support your true self.

One of the most important blessings of healing through compassionate and radical acceptance is the transition from external validation to internal value.

The midlife transition presents both obstacles and chances for personal growth. Although eating disorders are prevalent throughout this time of life, they don't have to define your experience. If you have expert help from practitioners who know the mental and physical aspects of recovery, you can move through this phase more easily and authentically. You can rethink your relationship with your body and life story by practicing awareness as well as acceptance, which will make room for real healing and a renewed sense of self.

Remember that aging does not have to be a condition of illness or alienation; regardless of where you are coming from, it can become a path of growing wisdom and self-discovery with the right support, loving awareness, and compassionate acceptance.

I want you to know that healing and recovery are NOT simply about the end of symptoms.

Here once again, is my take on recovery: It's not about weight, nor is it about food groups. It's highly nuanced. It's about understanding your true self and discovering your uniqueness. As I explained earlier, the definition of recovery is to regain what was lost or taken. Addiction, obsessive thoughts, and behaviors rob you of your ability to connect to the deepest part of yourself. Recovery, the healing I am referring to, allows for acceptance and understanding that every choice you've made, good, bad or ugly, was the best you could do at the time. You learn to accept your body size and shape rather than feel diminished by it. You learn to accept that eating is essential for life and living. You begin to accept the present moment and respond appropriately rather than numb or distract yourself from feelings or circumstances.

Reframing your belief system and letting go of the thoughts, feelings, and behaviors that, while once self-soothing, are no longer benefiting you allows you to create the fully nourished life you desire and deserve.

If you or anyone you know requires support or a higher level of care, here are a few resources for you to explore:

National Eating Disorders Association: https://www.nationaleatingdisorders.org

National Association of Anorexia Nervosa and Associated Disorders: https://anad.org/

Chapter Summary

This chapter addresses the often overlooked reality that eating disorders affect people across the lifespan, with midlife presenting unique challenges and triggers. We explore how significant life disruptions such as divorce, grief, care-giving responsibilities, hormonal shifts, empty nest transitions, and cultural messages about aging bodies can contribute to disordered eating patterns in midlife.

Personal Reflection Exercises

Exercise 1: Recognizing Midlife Triggers

This exercise helps identify which midlife-specific factors may be influencing your relationship with food:

1. **Review the following common midlife triggers for disordered eating:**

   - Significant relationship changes (divorce, loss, empty nest)

   - Care-giving responsibilities (for aging parents, children, grandchildren)

   - Hormonal transitions (perimenopause, menopause)

   - Identity shifts (career changes, retirement, children leaving home)

   - Body changes associated with aging

   - Financial pressures or transitions

   - Health diagnoses or concerns

2. **For each trigger that resonates with your experience:**

   - Rate its current impact on your life (1-10)

- Note specifically how it affects your relationship with food

- Identify what emotions arise in connection with this trigger

- Consider what needs might be seeking expression through food

3. **Compassionate Awareness:** Reflect on how understanding these triggers as normal life challenges rather than personal failings might shift your relationship with food behaviors. Write a self-compassionate message acknowledging the legitimate stressors you're navigating and how you're doing your best to cope.

- What emotion am I experiencing right now?

Exercise 2: Body Timeline Exploration

This exercise helps foster a broader perspective on your body's journey through life:

1. **Draw a timeline representing your life from childhood to the present.**

2. **Mark significant transitions and events along this timeline, both positive and challenging:**

- Developmental transitions (puberty, young adulthood, midlife)

- Major health events or changes

- Pregnancies or other physical experiences

- Times of significant body change

- Periods of disordered eating or body image distress

- Times of feeling at peace with your body

3. **For each period on your timeline, note:**

- What your body made possible for you during this time

- Challenges your body helped you navigate

- How your relationship with your body changed

4. **Looking at the timeline as a whole, reflect:**

- What patterns do you notice in your relationship with your body?

- How has your body shown resilience and wisdom throughout your life?

- What might it mean to honor your body's journey rather than resist it?

- What would radical acceptance of your body's entire journey look like?

This exercise helps expand your perspective beyond current struggles to see your body's whole journey–its wisdom, resilience, and capacity for healing.

Exercise 3: The Recovery Vision

This exercise helps you articulate what true recovery might look like beyond symptom management:

1. **Visioning Questions:** Take time to reflect deeply on these questions about what recovery means to you:

   - Beyond changes in food behaviors, what would recovery feel like in your daily life?

   - How would your relationship with your emotions transform?

   - What activities or connections might become more accessible?

   - How might your sense of identity expand beyond body concerns?

   - What values would guide your choices around food and body?

   - What forms of self-expression might emerge or

strengthen?

- How might your relationships change?

2. **Recovery Visualization:** Close your eyes and imagine yourself living in recovery. Create a detailed mental picture:

   - How do you start your day?

   - How do you respond to challenging emotions?

   - How do you experience meals and food?

   - How do you treat your body?

   - How do you engage with others?

   - What brings you joy and meaning?

3. **Recovery Letter:** Write a letter from your recovered self to your current self. Include:

   - Words of compassion for your current struggles

   - Insights about what truly matters

   - Guidance for the path ahead

   - Reminders of your inherent worthiness

   - Celebration of your courage in seeking healing

4. **Concrete Steps:** Identify three small, specific actions you could take this week that would align with your recovery vision. These might relate to food, emotional awareness, self-care, or connections with others.

Journal Prompts

1. **Beyond Symptoms:** I explain that "healing and recovery are NOT simply about the end of symptoms" and that true recovery is "highly nuanced...about the understanding of your true self, the discovery of your uniqueness." What might be possible in your life when healing extends beyond managing food behaviors? What aspects of your authentic self have been overshadowed by food and body preoccupation?

2. **Midlife Pressures:** The chapter describes how midlife brings unique pressures that can trigger or intensify disordered eating. Which midlife pressures have most affected your relationship with food and body? How might viewing these as normal life transitions rather than personal failures shift your perspective?

3. **Cultural Messages:** Reflect on the cultural messages about aging bodies that have influenced your relationship with your changing body. How have these messages created suffering? What alternative perspectives might offer

more peace and acceptance?

4. **Emotional Numbing:** The chapter explains how food behaviors often serve to numb or avoid difficult emotions. Which emotions do you find most challenging to feel fully? What were you taught about these emotions growing up? How might developing a different relationship with these emotions reduce your need for food as emotional management?

5. **Radical Acceptance:** Consider what radical acceptance of your midlife body might look like. How would your daily life change if you fully accepted your body's natural changes as part of your life journey rather than as problems to be fixed? What resistance arises when you contemplate this acceptance?

Practice: Creating a Personalized Recovery Toolkit

This practice helps you develop concrete tools for navigating challenging moments on your recovery journey:

Step 1: Identify Your Specific Challenges

Make a list of 3-5 specific challenging situations related to food, body image, or emotional regulation that you encounter regularly. For example:

- Feeling overwhelmed at the end of a workday

- Anxiety about social events involving food

- Negative body thoughts when getting dressed

- Comparison triggers on social media

- Stress from family care-giving responsibilities

Step 2: Create a Tool for Each Challenge

For each challenge, develop a specific, practical tool to help you respond with greater awareness and compassion. **For each tool, include:**

- A name that resonates with you

- When to use it (specific triggers or warning signs)

- Step-by-step instructions

- What you need (physical items, environment, support)

- How to adapt it for different settings

Example Tools:

- **The Pause Button:** A 60-second breathing practice for moments when stress triggers food urges

- **Body Gratitude Scan:** A brief meditation focusing on body function rather than appearance

- **Values Compass:** A quick check-in with core values to guide decisions in challenging moments

- **Emotion Naming:** A practice of specifically identifying and validating emotions before responding

- **Connection Reach:** A list of supportive people to contact when feeling isolated

Step 3: Create Access Points

Make these tools easily accessible in your daily life:

- Create digital notes on your phone

- Make small cards to keep in your purse or wallet

- Set reminders with tool names at triggering times of day

- Share tools with a trusted support person

- Practice regularly during less stressful times

Step 4: Implementation and Refinement

Commit to trying at least one tool daily for a week. After each use, briefly note:

- What triggered your need for the tool

- How effective it was in that moment

- How you might adapt it to be more helpful next time

Remember that recovery tools work best when practiced regularly. Start with small, consistent efforts rather than expecting perfection.

The Four Rs of Midlife Recovery Practice

This reflective practice builds on the concept of recovery as "regaining what was lost or taken" by focusing on four essential aspects of healing:

1. Reconnect: With Your Body's Wisdom

- Pause three times daily to check in with your body's sensations

- Ask: What physical sensations am I experiencing right now?

- Notice hunger, fullness, tension, ease, energy, fatigue without judgment

- Write down one thing you learned from your body's wisdom each day

2. Reclaim: Your Emotional Range

- Create an "emotion wheel" with the full spectrum of human emotions

- Each day, identify and name at least three emotions you experience

- For challenging emotions, practice saying: "I am feeling [emotion]. This is a normal human experience. I can be with this feeling with compassion."

- Explore connections between emotions and eating patterns with curiosity

3. Release: Perfectionism and Comparison

- Notice when perfectionist thoughts arise about food, body, or other areas

- Ask: Would I expect this level of perfection from someone I love?

- Practice "good enough" choices that honor both health and pleasure

- Create a media environment that supports recovery by curating social media feeds and other influences

4. Reimagine: Identity Beyond Body

- List aspects of your identity unrelated to appearance or food

- Engage weekly with one activity that nurtures these other dimensions

- Create affirmations that reflect your whole self: I am a person who...

- Visualize your life enriched by freedom from food and body preoccupation

Dedicate 5-10 minutes daily to focusing on one of these areas, rotating through all four each week. Record insights, challenges, and small victories in your recovery journal.

Compassionate Awareness Circle (Group Practice)

This practice creates a supportive space for exploring challenges and wisdom around midlife eating disorders:

Preparation:

- Gather 4-8 participants committed to respectful, confidential sharing

- Arrange chairs in a circle

- Provide a talking piece (a stone, feather, or other meaningful object)

- Designate a timekeeper

Opening (5 minutes):

- The facilitator welcomes participants and explains the circle format

- All participants take three collective breaths to center themselves

- The facilitator offers a brief reading on compassion or healing

Guidelines (5 minutes):

- Speak from personal experience using "I" statements

- Listen without interrupting or offering advice

- What is shared in the circle stays in the circle

- Participation in sharing is invited, not required

Round 1: Naming Our Experience (15-20 minutes) Pass the talking piece around the circle with the prompt: In one or two sentences, how would you describe your current relationship with food and your body?

Round 2: Exploring Wisdom (15-20 minutes) Pass the talking piece with the prompt: What has your journey with food and body taught you that might be valuable wisdom for your whole life?

Round 3: One Step Forward (15-20 minutes) Pass the talking piece with the prompt: What is one small, specific step you could take this week toward greater peace with food and body?

Closing (5 minutes):

- The facilitator acknowledges the courage it takes to engage in this work

- Participants offer one word that represents what they're taking from the circle

- The group takes three collective breaths to close the practice

This circle practice can be adapted for in-person or virtual meetings and repeated regularly as ongoing support for recovery.

Looking Forward

As you complete this section, remember that the path to recovery is not linear; it unfolds in spirals of growth, challenge, and deeper understanding. Each step toward greater awareness, each moment of compassion, each small act of honoring your body's wisdom contributes to your healing journey. Recovery in midlife offers unique opportunities for transformation. The very life transitions that can trigger disordered patterns also invite profound reassessment of what truly matters. As you navigate this threshold time, you bring decades of life experience, resilience, and wisdom to your healing process.

Remember my powerful assertion that true recovery extends far beyond symptom management to encompass "the understanding of your true self, the discovery of your uniqueness." This journey of reclaiming yourself is sacred work, worthy of your patience, commitment, and compassion.

Every day, remind yourself of this with these affirmations:

"I will accept my body size and shape rather than feel diminished by it."

"I accept that eating is essential for life and living."

"I accept the present moment and respond appropriately rather than numb or distract myself from feeling or circumstances."

"Healing and recovery are NOT simply about the end of symptoms ...It's about the understanding of your true self, the discovery of your uniqueness. – Mindy

Find Your Enough, Feel the Love, Face Your Feelings

The Invitation to Transformation

True healing begins with embracing uncomfortable truths and consciously choosing how you nourish both body and spirit. It's about facing your story with courage, understanding your unique biology, and transforming your mindset from within.

Your mindset is the gateway to lasting change. When you shift from scarcity—where fear and lack dominate your thoughts—to abundance, where love and gratitude guide your choices, you create space for profound transformation. This journey isn't about fixing your relationship with food first. Rather, when you reclaim your inherent worthiness, your relationship with food naturally evolves to reflect this newfound self-connection.

A New Foundation

In these pages, you'll discover how to create the foundation for what will become your newly transformed relationship with food, your body, your health, and ultimately, your life. Are you ready to stop fearing food and start celebrating its gifts? This path may feel unconventional but it leads to freedom, a freedom that allows you to release the hold diet culture has on you. Allow me to share where I was to illuminate the path.

My Journey Home

Each morning began the same way: my hands immediately traveled to my stomach, assessing its flatness, reaching for my hip bones to ensure they were prominent enough. The scale beckoned—a daily ritual that determined my mood, my worth, my entire day ahead. A "good" number ignited momentary elation; a "bad" number offered its own twisted comfort—permission to restrict, to control, to disappear, my safe place. I had surrendered my power to external validation, defining myself through what I imagined others saw. My inner voice insisted I needed to be thinner, smarter, somehow more of everything but less in physical form. For years, I believed I was fundamentally broken. My loving marriage and two remarkable daughters couldn't silence the persistent whisper that I simply wasn't enough, even though I'd raised them to be kind, generous, and successful.

Only when I embraced recovery–the process of reclaiming what was lost–did I recognize how much choice I actually had in how I responded to life's circumstances. I began to see life as a poker game: Sometimes you play the hand you're dealt, and sometimes you recognize when it's time to fold and wait for the next opportunity.

Cultivating gratitude required a profound mindset shift. I started simply by acknowledging my need for gratitude itself. Next came appreciation for the journey and my commitment to it, despite its challenges. What followed were monumental shifts as I opened myself to the love that had always surrounded me. I developed the courage to ask for the peace I longed for. The world's beauty revealed itself in ordinary moments like cloud formations, sunset colors, the rhythm of my breath.

My mind quieted, allowing me to relax into life's paradox: Amid uncertainty, everything was unfolding exactly as it should. Soon, what I expressed gratitude for manifested abundantly as I released the negativity that had held me captive.

Debi's Story: When "Not Enough" Becomes Your Identity

Debi sat across from me, her eyes reflecting both warmth and weariness. At sixty-two, she embodied the complexity of midlife, a woman with decades of wisdom and experience, yet felt somehow ungrounded as she navigated this new chapter.

As the middle child of three siblings, Debi carried beautiful memories of holiday tables surrounded by extended family—aunts bringing their signature dishes, her grandmother's hands skillfully crafting perfect pie crusts, her mother orchestrating it all with a kind of grace that seemed both effortless and extraordinary. Sunday dinners were sacred rituals in their home, where food was plentiful and lovingly prepared. These meals weren't merely about sustenance; they represented belonging, connection, tradition, and love that was tangible.

"Food was how we expressed everything in our family," Debi explained. "If you were celebrating, you celebrated with food. If you were grieving, you were comforted with food. If you achieved something remarkable, you were rewarded with something delicious. Food wasn't just nutrition; it was the language of our family's love."

This emotional blueprint established in childhood now shaped Debi's relationship with food as she navigates the complex terrain of her sixties. Her three children have established their homes, yet the invisible tethers of parenting remain firmly in place. Her eldest daughter was navigating a difficult divorce and often drops her children with Debi with little notice. Her son struggled with anxiety that periodically becomes debilitating, requiring her emotional support and presence. Her youngest daughter was building a career in another state but calls almost daily for guidance and reassurance.

"I love being needed," Debi admitted, "but occasionally I feel like I'm still putting everyone else first, just like I did when they were small. The difference is, back then I had a clear role. Now, I'm not sure who I am besides their mother."

This uncertainty extends beyond her family role. Before having children, Debi had been building a promising career in healthcare administration. What began as a temporary pause to raise her first child extended into nearly two decades away from her professional identity. When she attempted to return to the workforce in her late forties, the landscape had transformed dramatically. Technology had evolved, required credentials and experience had changed, and the confidence she once had eroded through years of focusing exclusively on others' needs.

"Sometimes I look back and wonder what might have been," she confessed. "Don't misunderstand, I cherish being a mother. But somewhere along the way, I lost parts of myself that had nothing to do with parenting. And now, I'm not sure how to reclaim them."

The sense of "not enough" permeates Debi's world—not accomplished enough professionally, not available enough for her adult children, not disciplined enough with her eating, not thin enough to feel comfortable in her body. This persistent feeling of inadequacy has created a painful cycle of seeking comfort in food and then feeling guilty and ashamed for doing so.

As a self-described "life-long dieter," Debi had internalized a framework that categorizes foods as either virtuous or villainous. This binary thinking—what many nutrition psychologists call

"all-or-nothing" thinking—had set her up for a persistent cycle of perceived failure.

Beyond Beautiful Words

Perhaps Debi's story resonates with thoughts and feelings you've pushed aside. My aim, however, isn't to offer inspiring words or captivating imagery; the internet overflows with these. Instead, I'm offering practical tools for lasting, sustainable transformation.

> **When we disengage from our inner critical voice and recognize it isn't the voice of truth, we free ourselves from the prison of our thoughts and fully inhabit our bodies.**

This reconnection is nothing short of magical—whether you consider it spiritual or simply energetic—as we tap into the wonder and intrinsic wisdom of the body we've been given.

We transform when we operate from love rather than fear, the fear of not being enough, the belief that our worth depends on a smaller physical presence. Love creates space for acceptance, compassion, and forgiveness. When we're truly present, love begins with ourselves. We live in gratitude, focusing on abundance rather than perceived lack, opening ourselves to the possibility that we can navigate whatever comes our way.

While this early concept forms the foundation of your journey to Food Freedom, it's simultaneously the ultimate destination.

Willingness vs. Willpower

I'm not asking you to surrender your power. Rather, I'm inviting you to reclaim it by disengaging from fear and limiting beliefs that perpetuate unhealthy patterns.

You already know that willpower doesn't work. It implies rigid control to restrain self-indulgence, which is a masculine approach fixated on results. Willingness, however, is a gentler state of being that prepares us to embrace change from a place of compassion, a feminine approach aligned with the journey itself. When our path includes self-kindness, we connect with the truth that has always resided within us. We reclaim what we forgot when we lost ourselves in food and negative body thoughts.

> **Your relationship with food mirrors your unique relationship with yourself and your story. Our stories differ, yet they've led us to the same place of fear and uncertainty.**

In our work together, Debi began to recognize that her association between food and comfort, love, and security, while rooted in beautiful family traditions, had evolved into a coping mechanism that no longer served her. The frequent episodes of losing herself in food had created not only physical discomfort but also a deeper emotional disconnection.

The consequences manifested physically in excess weight that strained her joints, digestive issues that disrupted her daily activities, skin breakouts that undermined her confidence, and unexplained inflammation that left her feeling perpetually fatigued. But perhaps more significantly, these patterns had created a mental landscape cluttered with food rules, self-judgment, and a pervasive sense of failure.

"I've been on every diet imaginable," she told me. "I've counted points, measured portions, eliminated entire food groups, tracked macros, fasted intermittently, and drunk my meals. I've lost the same thirty pounds at least a dozen times throughout my life. Each time I start over, I believe this time will be different. Each time I regain the weight, I feel like I've failed at the most basic aspect of self-control. I'll be 'good' for a while, then something stressful happens with one of the kids, and suddenly I'm standing in the kitchen at ten p.m., eating ice cream straight from the container. Then I hate myself for being so weak."

This narrative of personal failure represents one of the most pervasive and damaging aspects of diet culture. It places the responsibility for "success" or "failure" entirely on individual willpower, ignoring the biological, psychological, social, and cultural factors that influence our relationship with food.

Perhaps you believe you must handle everything alone, carrying burdens that require you to be bigger somehow. Maybe you feel undeserving when life offers goodness. Perhaps you fear losing someone's love if you change your appearance or behavior. The specifics matter less than the understanding that transforming your relationship with food isn't about becoming more or less of yourself, but becoming more authentically yourself.

When you lovingly transform your relationship with yourself, you transform your relationship with everything else.

The Gratitude Gateway

Gratitude awakens us to connection, with ourselves and others, like nothing else. It grounds us in the present moment and enables us to accept our beautiful imperfections. This acceptance creates an ease, a lightness of being that brings us home to ourselves.

Practicing gratitude addresses the two root causes of "not enough", the dissatisfaction and the compulsive pursuit of more to feel complete. We think, "If only I could lose this weight," "If only I exercised daily," "If only my partner communicated better," "If only I had more money..."

Gratitude's gift is that it reverses this outward-seeking pattern, immediately connecting us with the abundance already present in our lives.

For Debi, this seemed impossible at first.

"What do I have to be grateful for?" she asks, somewhat defensively. "My body hurts, my children still need constant support, and I've wasted decades trying to lose weight instead of building a career."

I invite her to start smaller, much smaller. "Can you find gratitude for the cup of tea you're holding right now? For the comfortable chair you're sitting in? For the fact that you're taking this time for yourself?"

Reluctantly, she began a daily gratitude practice, recording three things each morning for which she felt thankful. At first, her entries were perfunctory, such as "My house. My car. My family." But gradually, they became more specific and heartfelt, like "The way the morning light filters through my kitchen window. The depth of my grandson's laughter. The strength in my legs that will carry me through the grocery store today."

This simple practice began shifting her attention from what was missing to what was present, from scarcity to abundance. She hadn't changed her external circumstances, but she was gradually changing how she perceived them.

Gratitude secures us in the positive energy of NOW. Instead of postponing happiness until you lose those five, ten, or thirty pounds, gratitude for the journey brings joy to where you stand at this moment. You can wear beautiful clothes today, have that conversation with your boss about the raise you deserve, and express your needs to your partner.

Gratitude dissolves fear, revealing the loving-kindness essential for the nourished life you deserve. This transformative practice is woven into many spiritual traditions. In Jewish practice, the first morning prayer expresses gratitude: "I am grateful. Thank you for returning my soul to me with enormous compassion." Buddhist practice begins each day acknowledging the precious gift of human life and its impermanent nature, asking, "How shall I live this precious day? What deserves my attention today?"

Even science confirms gratitude's power. Research has documented gratitude as an attitude, mood, and emotion with profound effects. Studies indicate that weekly gratitude journaling increases overall well-being—participants exercised more, slept better, enjoyed improved health, and maintained a more optimistic outlook.[1] Even a single expression of thoughtful gratitude produces immediate increases in happiness and decreases in depressive symptoms, with consistent practice yielding lasting positive results.

A heart filled with gratitude generates actions that complete the circle between gifts offered,

---

1. Emmons, R. A., & McCullough, M. E. (2003). Counting blessings versus burdens: An experimental investigation of gratitude and subjective well-being in daily life. Journal of Personality and Social Psychology, 84(2), 377-389. https://doi.org/10.1037/0022-3514.84.2.377

our willingness to receive, and their universal source.

The Courage to Feel

When I asked Debi what emotions typically preceded her episodes of nighttime eating, she paused. "I don't know," she finally admitted. "I just know I feel bad, and then I'm standing in front of the refrigerator."

This disconnection from specific emotions is common among those who've used food to numb uncomfortable feelings. Over time, the pattern becomes so automatic that we bypass conscious awareness of the emotion itself, moving directly from discomfort to the behavior that temporarily soothes it.

Our work together focused on creating a pause, a moment of awareness between feeling and action. I asked her to keep a simple journal next to her bed, recording instances when she felt drawn to eat outside of mealtimes. Before eating anything, she would write down what she was feeling at that moment.

The first week's entries were sparse: "Stressed." "Tired." "Annoyed." But as she continued the practice, she could pinpoint her emotions more specifically: "Disappointed that my daughter canceled our lunch plans again." "Angry that my ex-husband still hasn't increased his support payments despite promising to do so." "Lonely in this empty house after years of constant activity."

Facing our feelings can terrify us. When you've turned to compulsive behaviors to numb uncomfortable emotions, it was a brilliant survival strategy at the time. Numbing, any activity that desensitizes feelings to avoid vulnerability, protected you then. It prevented you from confronting these feelings and realizing they weren't scary.

Consider where your stories began. Were they responses to someone else's wounding? Can you find compassion for their origins? Many of us heard messages like "Stop crying or I'll give you something to cry about" or "Do as I say, not as I do." These messages implied that we shouldn't feel the need to be ourselves. Likely, those who delivered these messages received them themselves. Once we bring awareness and questioning to these narratives, we often discover they no longer serve us.

For Debi, this exploration revealed that her mother's approach to emotions had profoundly shaped her own. "My mother was from that generation that believed in keeping up appearances," she recalled. "She would say, 'No one wants to hear about your problems,' or 'Pull yourself together.' I learned early that difficult emotions should be managed privately, preferably with something sweet to take the edge off."

This insight helped Debi approach her eating in response to emotionally charged situations with compassion rather than judgment. She wasn't weak or broken; she was applying coping strategies she'd learned in childhood. With this understanding, she could begin developing new responses to her emotions—responses that honored rather than suppressed her feelings.

Accepting what you cannot change while facing what you can creates space for forgiveness and tremendous growth.

Through this process, you begin experiencing loving-kindness and compassion. Compassion leads to forgiveness and releases the struggle with what was. Forgiveness lets go of judgment, anger, and ultimately, fear. When you're forgiving and compassionate, nourishment flows from within. This perspective reveals your attachment to your story and gently guides you to release it. While your story remains yours, how you relate to it determines whether you can write your own "happily ever after."

As author Melody Beattie teaches, when we identify the problem and feel the feelings, we redirect our life's course.[2] Be grateful for everything—the blessing is in feeling it, being humbled by it, and letting go of what no longer serves you.

Emotions become feelings, which become thoughts that solidify into beliefs. It's easy to surrender your power to them as they gain momentum. When you realize feelings are just feelings and thoughts are just thoughts—not facts, not your identity—you can meet them, experience them, process them, and release them.

---

2. Beattie, Melody. *Codependent No More: How to Stop Controlling Others and Start Caring for Yourself.* Hazelden Publishing, 2022.

Not feeling means checking out; numbing disconnects us not only from difficult emotions but also from life's goodness.

When we face feelings, embrace them, and move through them, we reclaim our power.

Deprivation and Nourishment

A pivotal moment in Debi's journey occurred when she recognized that choosing foods that support her well-being isn't an act of restriction but an expression of self-respect. This subtle yet profound shift in perspective transformed how she approaches eating.

"I'm learning that choosing not to eat something that doesn't serve me doesn't mean I'm restricting, it means I'm making an empowered choice to stand in my value as I honor my body's wisdom," she explained. "When I consider how certain foods affect my digestion, my energy, my sleep, and my mood, I'm acknowledging that my body deserves care and consideration."

This framework moves beyond the simplistic good food/bad food dialogue that had governed her relationship with eating. Instead, it introduces nuance: How does this particular food make me feel? How does it affect my energy? My digestion? My sleep? My mood? This curiosity creates space for personalization rather than adherence to external rules.

Through this approach, Debi discovered that certain foods she previously considered comfort foods actually create significant physical discomfort. The pasta dishes she associates with her mother's love leave her feeling bloated and lethargic. The baked goods that remind her of childhood celebrations trigger inflammatory responses that manifest as joint pain and skin eruptions.

Simultaneously, she discovered that foods she had previously categorized as "diet foods" or "healthy but boring" options can be prepared in ways that provide both physical nourishment and emotional satisfaction. The process of cooking became meditative, as well as creative. The vibrant colors on her plate brought visual pleasure. The complex flavors engaged her senses fully.

Most importantly, she began to recognize when she approached food from a place of self-care versus self-soothing. This awareness didn't eliminate her desire for emotional eating, but it created a pause—a moment of choice where she can ask herself what she truly needs in that moment.

I've explained that her pull to indulge in an effort not to feel deprived actually created the ultimate deprivation; it distanced her from creating the life she truly wants. Since she associated food with comfort, love, and security, losing herself to frequent binges had become routine.

The challenge we worked on was to replace Debi's comfort foods with those that calmed her body's inflammatory response as well as managed her anxiety. She learned to nourish herself with nutrients and foods that are emotionally satisfying yet not disruptive to her system.

The limiting beliefs that hold us back are rooted in fear. "Afraid" comes from "frai," meaning "beloved, precious, at peace," with the prefix "a" meaning "away from." Thus, afraid literally means being away from feeling beloved, precious, and at peace. Fear disrupts our equilibrium, triggering stress physiology and disconnecting us from our body's wisdom. While fear's survival mechanisms serve us when facing genuine threats, often what we fear is merely a perceived danger—a reaction to beliefs we've constructed.

All promises to self and commitments to loved ones will meet resistance until you release attachment to false beliefs about yourself and food.

How many unfulfilled promises weigh on you? This mental burden manifests as excess baggage that eventually depletes you.

Letting go creates the lightness of being. When you feel lighter, you become lighter. When you're FREE, you make changes from within, naturally transforming your outer reality.

The Power of Love

As Brené Brown writes, "We cultivate love when we allow our most vulnerable and powerful selves to be deeply seen and known, and when we honor the spiritual connection that grows from offering trust, respect, kindness, and affection." In other words, love is the most powerful force we know—what we're all ultimately seeking. To find it, we must first offer it to ourselves, which can be hard when feeling unworthy or burdened by past beliefs. Adding love to your emotional landscape means freeing yourself from attachment to a past with no future and experiencing peace and preciousness in the present. As you cultivate self-love, find compassion for different chapters of your story. What would you say now to your awkward, confused teenage self? How would you respond with compassion to times when fear caused you to push others away? Compassion allows you to see with wholeness and eyes wide open.[3]

Even in our darkest moments, we possess the power to choose love over fear, opening life to new dimensions.

Debi was willing to look at what she needed in order to be nourished outside of the kitchen, away from the dining table, for we're nourished by so much more than the food on our plates. (More on this in Chapter 9.) The essential nourishment we crave is available through our relationships, our purpose, and the spirituality that calls to us. We are nourished by the experiences that surround us and the lifestyle choices we make, which are influenced by how well we sleep and how often we appropriately move. And when it comes to food, the heartiness and sentiment of that meal are nourishing as well.

In Debi's case, and maybe yours too, it's important to remember to honor this part of the story, the feast that is your life. At the

---

3. Brown, Brené. The Gifts of Imperfection: Let Go of Who You Think You're Supposed to Be and Embrace Who You Are. Hazelden Publishing, 2010.

same time, the intention you bring with you to the table speaks to WHO you are as an eater. The consciousness that transforms Debi's eating naturally influenced how she engaged with her adult children, how she explored new interests, how she related to her changing body, and how she envisioned her future.

The love I'm describing isn't romantic—it's a love that fills you with serene joy. Once experienced, it connects you to your essence, which needs no distraction. You stop obsessing about thinness and discover being without judgment. You finally come home to yourself, heart full.

How do I know this? After many years journeying homeward, I feel grounded at last. Recently, hand in hand with my husband, I strolled along the beach during our winter escape. The sky shone robin's-egg blue, the water felt perfect, and the gentle breeze embraced us like a warm hug. In that moment came a new and novel awareness; I was in love with myself. I walked in my swimsuit without worrying about my thighs, belly, what I'd eaten, what dinner would be, or how I compared to the younger bodies nearby. Simply making footprints in the sand was enough to make me feel complete.

Finding our enough, feeling the love, and facing our feelings reveals that we're ready to shine brilliantly, through life's inevitable highs and lows, allowing us to return home as our most radiant, authentic selves.

Chapter Summary

In this chapter, we explore the core elements of midlife healing: finding our sense of "enough," cultivating self-love, and facing our emotions rather than numbing them with food as the foundation for food freedom. Through Debi's story of lifelong dieting and the associations she formed between food, love, and comfort in childhood, we see how emotional patterns established early in life can shape our relationship with food decades later.

The chapter also introduces the power of gratitude to shift us from the mindset of scarcity to one of abundance, the importance of creating space between emotions and actions, and the paradigm shift from seeing food choices as restriction to viewing them as empowered acts of self-care. Now you can discover how transforming your relationship with yourself naturally transforms your relationship with food, illustrating this truth through my personal journey toward self-acceptance and embodied peace.

Personal Reflection Exercises

Exercise 1: Exploring Your "Not Enough" Stories

Reflect on the areas of your life where you experience the "not enough" feeling that Debi described:

- Draw a circle in the center of a page and write "I am enough" inside it.

- Around this circle, create branches for different areas where you sometimes feel inadequate (body, career, motherhood, relationships, etc.).

- For each branch, write down the specific "not enough" messages you tell yourself.

- Next to each message, note when you first remember hearing or developing this belief. Was it from family, media, a specific experience, or comparison with others?

Now, revisit each "not enough" message and write a compassionate counter-narrative that acknowledges your wholeness and value beyond these limiting beliefs.

Exercise 2: Gratitude Gateway Practice

For one week, practice this three-part gratitude ritual:

Morning: Before getting out of bed, place your hand on your heart and name three things you're grateful for at this moment.

Throughout the day: Set three specific times (perhaps meal times) to pause and acknowledge something you're grateful for in your body, regardless of its size or appearance. For example: "I'm grateful for my legs that carried me through my errands today," or "I'm grateful for my hands that allow me to create and connect."

Evening: Before sleep, write down:

- One moment from the day when you felt enough just as you are

- One way you showed yourself compassion today

- One thing you're looking forward to tomorrow

At the end of the week, reflect: How has this practice affected your thought patterns around food and body? What shifts have you noticed in your emotional landscape? How has gratitude influenced your sense of enough-ness?

Journal Prompts

1. **Willingness vs. Willpower:** I describe willpower as "rigid control to restrain self-indulgence while willingness is "a gentler state of being that prepares us to embrace change from a place of compassion." Reflect on times when you've approached food changes from willpower versus willingness. How did these approaches feel differ-

ent? What results did they produce?

2. **Emotional Eating Awareness:** Think about a recent instance when you turned to food for comfort or distraction. Can you identify what you were feeling beforehand? What would have happened if you had allowed yourself to fully experience that emotion instead? What might you have needed at that moment besides food?

3. **Food as Language:** Debi shared how in her family, "Food was how we expressed everything." How was food used to express love, celebration, comfort, or other emotions in your family of origin? How has this emotional blueprint influenced your current relationship with food?

4. **Self-Compassion Practice:** Reflect on this: What would you say now to your awkward, confused teenage self? Write a letter to your younger self about her relationship with food and body, offering the wisdom and compassion you've gained through your life experience.

5. **Being vs. Becoming:** Reflect on my beach experience when I realized I was in love with myself. Imagine a similar moment of complete self-acceptance for yourself. What would you be doing? Who would be with you? What thoughts about food or your body would be absent? How would this freedom feel in your body?

Practice: Creating the Pause

This week, practice creating a pause between emotional triggers and food responses:

1. **Identify Your Triggers**: Notice patterns of when you're most likely to turn to food for comfort (certain times of day, after specific interactions, during particular emotional states).

2. **Place Visual Reminders**: Put small symbols or notes in places where emotional eating typically occurs (kitchen, pantry, desk drawer, car) to remind you to pause.

3. **Practice the PAUSE Technique**:

   ○ **P - Pause**: Stop and take a full breath

   ○ **A - Awareness:** Notice what you're feeling physically and emotionally

   ○ **U - Understand**: Ask, "What am I really needing right now?"

   ○ **S - Select**: Choose a response that truly addresses this need

   ○ **E - Evaluate**: After responding, notice how you feel

4. **Create an Emotional Needs Menu**:
List non-food ways to address common emotional needs

- For comfort: warm bath, soft blanket, calming music, gentle movement

- For stimulation: walk outside, energizing music, call a friend, creative project

- For distraction: short meditation, reading, puzzle, craft activity

- For celebration: text a friend, journal the achievement, create a ritual

- For connection: reach out to someone, engage with a pet, connect with nature

Remember, sometimes food will still be the appropriate response, and that's perfectly okay. The goal isn't to never eat emotionally but to expand your repertoire of emotional care beyond food alone.

Looking Forward

As we close this chapter on finding your enough, feeling the love, and facing your feelings, remember that this journey isn't about perfection—it's about presence. When you choose to meet yourself with curiosity rather than criticism, when you honor your emotions as messengers rather than enemies, and when you recognize that true nourishment extends far beyond your plate, you create the foundation for lasting transformation. The path to food freedom begins not with another set of rules, but with the radical act of coming home to yourself.

"The most profound shift happens when you realize that healing isn't about becoming someone new—it's about remembering who you've always been beneath the layers of 'not enough.' When you finally see yourself through the eyes of love rather than judgment, everything else naturally falls into place, including your relationship with food."
—Mindy

The Mind-Body-Gut Connection

Stress, Hormones, and Your Relationship with Food

Breaking Free from the Stress-Food Cycle

If you've opened these pages, you're likely seeking to transform how you relate to food and your body. The journey toward healing begins with understanding a profound truth: Your relationship with food often mirrors your more profound relationship with yourself and your life experiences. I know; I am repeating myself! But when we approach this relationship through the lens of functional medicine, we see not just behaviors but the intricate web of biochemical, hormonal, and neurological influences that shape them.

The interplay between stress and a disordered relationship with eating creates a complex cycle that can feel impossible to break. Feelings of overwhelm may trigger restrictive or binge-eating behaviors as coping mechanisms. For those who restrict, the illusion of control provides temporary relief from life's uncertainties. For those who binge, there's momentary comfort and emotional numbing—a brief reprieve from pain or anxiety. Yet these behaviors, while offering fleeting escape, ultimately amplify both physical and psychological stress, creating a self-perpetuating cycle that becomes increasingly difficult to escape with each cycle.

This issue is not about willpower—it's about biology, psychology, and the body's innate wisdom. Your path toward transformative healing requires honoring this wisdom rather than fighting against it.

The Symphony of Stress Response

From a functional medicine perspective, stress manifests as a sophisticated biochemical cascade throughout your entire body. This response evolved as a survival adaptation, your body's brilliant way of protecting you from danger.

When faced with a stressor, be it physical danger or emotional distress, your body initiates a complex series of reactions. Blood rushes to your limbs, your heart rate and blood pressure increase, and stress hormones like cortisol and adrenaline flood your system. Blood flow redirects to your brain for quick thinking. Glucose is released into your bloodstream for immediate energy. Your muscles tense, preparing for action. All of this occurs within minutes, sometimes seconds, preparing you to respond effectively to the perceived threat.

In ancestral environments, this response was life-saving, enabling our fore-mothers to escape predators, protect their children, and navigate environmental challenges. Today, this same exquisite system can be activated by work deadlines, relationship challenges, financial worries, social media comparisons, and—significantly—by our thoughts about food and body image. When stress becomes chronic, this elegant survival system transforms into a source of imbalance, undermining the very health it evolved to protect.

Consider for a moment how often throughout your day your body receives signals of threat. An alarm jolts you awake. The news headlines can evoke anxiety even before you've had breakfast. The traffic raises your blood pressure. The critical inner voice accompanies your reflection in the mirror. The endless to-do list that never quite gets completed. Each of these moments may trigger subtle or pronounced stress responses, creating a physiological state that profoundly affects your relationship with food and your body.

Your Second Brain: The Gut-Brain Connection

Your central nervous system and metabolism are deeply interconnected, and nowhere is their relationship more evident than in
what Johns Hopkins Medical Center refers to as your "second
brain,"the Enteric Nervous System (ENS). This remarkable net-
work consists of two thin layers of over one-hundred-million nerve
cells lining your digestive tract from esophagus to rectum.[1]

The ENS controls crucial digestive functions, including:

- Swallowing

- The release of digestive enzymes

- Nutrient absorption

- Blood flow throughout the digestive system

- Elimination of waste

**This "brain in your gut" communicates bidi-
rectionally with your central nervous system,
creating what functional medicine practitioners
recognize as the gut-brain axis. This connectivi-
ty is not just metaphorical, it's a physical reality.**

---

1. Johns Hopkins Medicine. "The Brain-Gut Connection." Johns Hopkins Medicine, accessed
2024. https://www.hopkinsmedicine.org/health/wellness-a
nd-prevention/the-brain-gut-connection

The vagus nerve, the longest cranial nerve in your body, serves as the primary communication channel between your gut and brain, transmitting information about emotional states to your digestive system and sending messages about digestive conditions back to your brain. When this communication becomes disrupted, the effects can manifest throughout your body.

The Autonomic Nervous System (ANS)—which regulates digestive function—operates through two primary channels:

- The parasympathetic nervous system: Your "rest and digest" mode; when digestion is optimized, stress hormones are low, and your body can assimilate nutrients effectively.

- The sympathetic nervous system: Your "fight or flight" mode; when digestion slows, stress hormones rise, and the body prioritizes immediate survival over nourishment

When you eat in a stressed state—rushing through meals, multitasking, scrolling through disturbing news, arguing, or consumed by guilt about food choices—you're asking your body to perform contradictory functions.

You're providing nourishment while simultaneously signaling danger. This contradiction creates a physiological conflict that can manifest as digestive distress, diminished nutrient absorption, and disrupted hunger and fullness cues.

Your Gut Microbiome: The Foundation of Health

Your digestive tract houses approximately one-hundred-trillion microorganisms, more bacteria than there are cells in your entire body.

This ecosystem, known as your microbiome, plays a critical role in:

- Digesting food
- Absorbing and manufacturing nutrients
- Breaking down medications
- Supporting immune function (eighty percent of your immune system resides in your gut)
- Regulating mood and cognitive function
- Protecting against harmful pathogens
- Reducing inflammation
- Contributing to hormonal balance

When this delicate balance of microorganisms is disrupted—a condition called dysbiosis—it can trigger a cascade of effects throughout your body. Research increasingly connects gut dysbiosis with conditions including:

- Digestive disorders (IBS, IBD, GERD, SIBO)
- Mood imbalances (anxiety, depression)
- Autoimmune conditions
- Skin issues (eczema, psoriasis, acne, rosacea)
- Hormonal imbalances

- Weight management difficulties

- Chronic fatigue

- Brain fog and cognitive challenges

- Food sensitivities and allergies

This connection explains why improving gut health often leads to improvements in seemingly unrelated areas of health. When we address the foundation, the entire structure becomes more stable.

In my practice, I've witnessed women who've struggled for decades with anxiety or depression experience remarkable improvements when we focus on healing their gut microbiome. Similarly, many who've battled weight fluctuations discover that balancing their gut ecology creates a more stable metabolic environment that supports their body's natural weight regulation.

The Gut-Brain-Hormone Connection in Midlife

This mind-body-gut connection becomes even more significant during hormonal transitions of midlife. As estrogen and progesterone levels fluctuate and eventually decline, the body becomes increasingly sensitive to stress. Many women notice changes in digestive function, stress resilience, and metabolic response during perimenopause and menopause.

Your gut microbiome influences and is influenced by your hormonal balance. Estrogen levels, in particular, have a bidirectional relationship with gut health:[2]

- Estrogen affects gut permeability: Declining estrogen can alter the integrity of the intestinal barrier, potentially increasing inflammation and affecting neurotransmitter production.[3]

- Gut bacteria regulate estrogen: Certain gut bacteria contain an enzyme called beta-glucuronidase, which affects how estrogen is metabolized and recirculated in the body. Dysbiosis can lead to improper estrogen metabolism, exacerbating hormonal imbalances.[4]

- Neurotransmitter production: Approximately ninety-five percent of serotonin—your "happiness" neurotransmitter—is produced in the gut. Gut dysbiosis can disrupt this production, significantly affecting mood, appetite regulation, and stress response.

During midlife transitions, this intricate relationship becomes particularly relevant. The hormonal fluctuations characteristic of perimenopause can trigger digestive symptoms (bloating, constipation, food sensitivities) that weren't previously present. Simul-

---

2. https://www.frontiersin.org/journals/microbiology/articles/10.3389/fmicb.2021.711137/full

3. https://www.mdpi.com/1422-0067/24/16/12822

4. https://www.maturitas.org/article/S0378-5122(17)30650-3/fulltext

taneously, gut health changes can intensify hormonal symptoms like hot flashes, mood swings, and sleep disturbances.

I've worked with countless women who initially sought support for symptoms they didn't realize were connected such as the late-night chocolate cravings alongside sleep disruptions, the new digestive sensitivities alongside mood fluctuations, the seemingly sudden weight changes despite maintaining similar eating patterns. When we address these symptoms through the lens of the gut-brain-hormone connection, we can create comprehensive healing that honors the body's collective wisdom.

The Hormonal Symphony of Stress and Weight

From a functional medicine perspective, chronic stress creates a cascade of hormonal imbalances that directly impact weight management:

- Cortisol: Often called the "stress hormone," cortisol signals the body to store fat, particularly around the abdomen. This visceral fat isn't merely aesthetic, it's metabolically active tissue that produces inflammatory compounds and can further disrupt hormonal balance. In midlife, when estrogen's protective effect diminishes, cortisol's impact becomes even more pronounced.

- Insulin: Stress triggers insulin release, which removes glucose from the bloodstream. Chronically elevated insulin promotes fat storage and blocks fat burning. This becomes even more pronounced during the insulin resistance that often accompanies midlife hormonal shifts. Many women find that foods they've enjoyed without difficulty throughout their lives suddenly trigger blood sugar imbalances during perimenopause.

- Ghrelin and Leptin: These hunger-regulating hormones become dysregulated under chronic stress. Ghrelin (which stimulates appetite) increases while leptin (which signals fullness) becomes less effective, leading to increased hunger and diminished satiety. This dysregulation can create confusing hunger signals that disconnect you from your body's true needs.

- Thyroid Hormones: Stress can suppress thyroid function, slowing metabolism and energy production throughout the body. Many women experience subtle thyroid imbalances during midlife transitions that contribute to fatigue, cold intolerance, and weight management challenges.

When you add the neurobiological factor—that high-sugar, high-fat foods temporarily reduce stress hormone production by activating pleasure centers in the brain—you can see why eating to self-soothe becomes such a powerful coping strategy. Your body isn't betraying you; it's attempting to find balance within challenging circumstances.

Midlife Metabolic Changes Through a Functional Lens

As women transition through perimenopause and menopause, metabolic flexibility often decreases. The body becomes less efficient at switching between carbohydrate and fat burning, making weight management more challenging. Additionally, declining estrogen affects:

- Fat distribution (shifting toward abdominal storage)

- Insulin sensitivity (increasing risk of insulin resistance)

- Sleep quality (disrupting hunger hormones and stress regulation)

- Gut microbiome diversity (affecting nutrient absorption and inflammation)

- Energy expenditure (decreasing baseline caloric needs)

- Muscle mass (reducing metabolic activity without resistance training)

- Satiety hormones (altering hunger and fullness signals)

These changes aren't signs that your body is betraying you; they're adaptations requiring a more nuanced approach to nourishment and self-care. Understanding these processes allows you to work with your body's changing needs rather than fighting against them.

One client, Marla, came to me frustrated after gaining fifteen pounds despite maintaining her lifelong eating and exercise patterns. She'd been told by previous practitioners that weight gain was simply an inevitable part of aging that she should accept. While I believe in radical acceptance of our bodies at every stage, I also know that understanding the physiological changes occurring during midlife transitions requires us to adapt consciously. By addressing Marla's gut health, optimizing her protein intake, introducing specific resistance training, and teaching stress-reduction techniques, she found a new equilibrium that honored her body's changing needs while supporting her goals and well-being.

The Physical Impact of Chronic Stress on Digestion

The effects of prolonged, low-level stress on digestive function are profound:

- Decreased blood flow to your digestive tract (up to four times less)

- A twenty-thousand-fold decrease in digestive enzyme production

- Increased digestive distress (heartburn, bloating, gas, constipation, diarrhea)

- Reduced beneficial gut bacteria

- Intestinal permeability (leaky gut)

- Excretion of essential minerals like calcium and magnesium

- Decreased absorption of water-soluble vitamins (B and C)

- Reduced oxygen uptake in the digestive tract

- Increased systemic inflammation

- Decreased calorie-burning efficiency

- Altered gut motility (either slowing or accelerating transit time)

- Disruption of the microbiome's daily rhythms

Even if you're consuming the most nutrient-dense foods available, eating in a stressed state dramatically reduces their beneficial im-

pact. The solution isn't just changing what you eat—it's transforming how you eat and, more fundamentally, how you relate to the act of nourishing yourself.

Consider this: How often do you eat while truly relaxed, present, and grateful? How frequently do meals become another task to complete while simultaneously responding to emails, managing family logistics, or consuming troubling news? The state of your nervous system during eating may be as important as the nutritional content of your meal.

The Wisdom of Relaxed Eating

Do you remember the French Paradox? This is the observation that French culture embraces pleasure in eating without the corresponding rates of obesity seen in other Western nations. Beyond the nutritional composition of their meals lies something equally powerful: their relationship with food.

Traditional French eating habits prioritize:
- Presence and pleasure during meals
- Unhurried eating in relaxed settings
- Social connection and conversation
- Appreciation for quality over quantity
- Midday emphasis for larger meals when digestion is optimized
- Clear delineation between meal times and other activities
- Mindful enjoyment of indulgent foods in appropriate portions

- Seasonal, local, and diverse food choices

- Minimal snacking between meals

So remember that when we eat in a parasympathetic (relaxed) state, our bodies:

- Increase digestive enzyme production by up to twenty-thou-sand-fold

- Optimize nutrient absorption

- Support healthy gut bacteria

- Balance blood sugar response

- Enhance metabolic efficiency

- Recognize satiety signals more effectively

- Reduce inflammation

- Strengthen the mind-body connection

- Create positive associations with nourishment

Have you ever noticed returning from vacation actually lighter despite eating more freely? This paradox illustrates how powerful-ly stress reduction influences metabolism and digestion. When we release the anxiety, guilt, and hypervigilance around food, we often discover our body's natural regulatory wisdom.

One client, Jennifer, meticulously tracked every calorie for years yet struggled with persistent digestive issues and weight fluctua-tions. During a two-week vacation in Italy, she allowed herself to eat pasta, enjoy local wines, and savor gelato—without her track-ing app. To her surprise, she returned home feeling better in her body than she had in years, with improved digestion and stable energy. The difference wasn't what she ate but how she ate it, with pleasure, presence, and without the constant stress of monitoring and judgment.

Three Steps to Nourish Your Gut-Brain Connection**

1. Cultivate Beneficial Gut Bacteria

Your microbiome thrives on diversity and balance. Here's how to support your beneficial bacteria:

Introduce probiotic-rich foods and supplements:

- Live-culture yogurt (unsweetened)
- Kefir
- Unpasteurized cheeses (Gouda, Cheddar, Provolone)
- Fermented vegetables (sauerkraut, kimchi)
- Miso
- Kombucha
- Apple cider vinegar
- Tempeh
- Beet

Feed your beneficial bacteria with prebiotic foods:

- Garlic and onions
- Jerusalem artichokes
- Dandelion greens
- Asparagus
- Bananas (especially slightly underripe)
- Oats
- Flaxseeds
- Apples

- Jicama
- Chicory root
- Leeks

Consider targeted supplementation:

- Specialized probiotic strains based on your specific needs
- Prebiotic fibers like inulin or resistant starches
- L-glutamine for intestinal lining support
- Omega-3 fatty acids for reducing inflammation
- Digestive enzymes when appropriate

**Please consult your healthcare team before adding supplementation, and if you are suffering from digestive symptoms, it is a beneficial idea to work with a practitioner before adding certain foods.

2. Reduce Stress, Increase Joy

Chronic stress directly impacts your gut microbiome. Research shows that prolonged stress can alter the composition and function of gut bacteria, potentially leading to increased intestinal permeability and inflammation.

Remarkably, positive emotions can have the opposite effect. Incorporate daily practices that activate your parasympathetic nervous system:

- Conscious breathing exercises (even two minutes makes a difference)
- Mindfulness meditation
- Time in nature
- Laughter and play

- Gentle movement

- Creative expression

- Connection with loved ones

- Gratitude practices

- Sensory pleasure (aromatherapy, music, touch)

- Progressive muscle relaxation

- Guided imagery

- Yoga

- Forest bathing

- Tai chi or qigong

Create rituals that signal safety to your nervous system:

- A morning routine that grounds you before engaging with technology

- A designated "worry time" that compartmentalizes anxious thoughts

- Technology boundaries that protect your nervous system

- Transition rituals between work and home life

- Evening practices that prepare your body for restful sleep

3. Embrace Nature's Wisdom

Our modern obsession with anti-bacterial may be contributing to gut dysbiosis. The "hygiene hypothesis" suggests that our reduced exposure to beneficial microorganisms may be contributing to increased allergies, autoimmune conditions, and inflammatory disorders.

Consider:

- Spending time in natural environments

- Gardening (soil contains beneficial microorganisms)
- Reducing use of antibacterial products
- Sharing your home with pets (they safely expose us to beneficial bacteria)
- Embracing occasional "messiness" in your environment
- Choosing organic produce when possible (soil microbiome diversity)
- Harvesting wild foods when safe and available
- Swimming in natural bodies of water
- Walking barefoot on natural surfaces
- Diversifying your food sources and preparation methods

Cultivating Resilience Through Functional Medicine

Resilience, the capacity to recover from difficulties, becomes the foundation for healing your relationship with food and body. From a functional medicine perspective, resilience isn't merely psychological; it's physiological, supported by:

- Optimized gut health: Supporting diverse microbiome populations that influence mood, stress response, and inflammation
- Balanced blood sugar: Stabilizing energy and reducing stress-driven cravings
- Adequate micronutrients: Providing the building blocks for neurotransmitters and stress-adaptation hormones
- Quality sleep: Allowing the nervous system to regulate and stress hormones to reset

- Mindful movement: Reducing inflammation and supporting stress hormone balance

- Social connection: Activating oxytocin and other bonding hormones that counter stress

- Present-moment awareness: Training the nervous system to distinguish between genuine threats and habitual stress responses

- Hydration: Supporting cellular function and detoxification pathways

- Exposure to natural light: Regulating circadian rhythms and vitamin D production

- Detoxification support: Reducing toxic burden on your body's systems

Each of these elements contributes to your body's capacity to maintain balance amidst life's inevitable changes and challenges. By strengthening these foundations, you create a physiological environment that supports healing in your relationship with food and body.

The Path Forward: Relaxing Into Wholeness

Healing your relationship with food means honoring the wisdom of your body rather than fighting against it. The path forward isn't found through more rigid control or deprivation, but through cultivating presence, compassion, and physiological balance.

When we release the stress about what food will "do to us," we create space for food to nourish us

fully. When we eat while relaxed, truly present with our food and our bodies, we access the body's innate capacity for self-regulation.

Every meal becomes an opportunity to practice this relaxation response:

Remember that oxygen is a fundamental nutrient. Deep, rhythmic breathing signals safety to your nervous system, optimizing digestion and metabolic function. This simple practice can transform your relationship with food and your body.

Embracing the Journey

Changing your relationship with food is more than changing what's on your plate; it's about how you show up at the table. It's about nourishing not just your physical body but your whole being.

The journey isn't always linear. There will be moments when old patterns emerge, especially during times of stress or hormonal fluctuation. Approach these moments with curiosity rather than judgment, asking, "What is my body trying to tell me? What do I truly need right now?"

By understanding the intricate dance between stress, gut health, hormones, and eating behaviors, you gain the power to create new patterns. You begin to recognize that worrying about weight often increases weight, while relaxing into nourishment allows your body to find its natural balance.

This is your invitation to restore harmony with food, to count blessings over calories, and to understand that genuine nourishment extends beyond the nutrients on your plate. It's about creating a life that feeds your soul as well as your body.

One client beautifully expressed her transformation. "For decades, I viewed my body as a problem to be solved. Now I see it as wisdom to be honored. This shift hasn't just changed my relationship with food, it's changed my relationship with life itself."

Practice: Cultivating the Relaxation Response

Conscious Breathing: Place the tip of your tongue just behind your upper front teeth. Exhale completely through your mouth. Close your mouth and inhale quietly through your nose for a count of four. Hold your breath for a count of seven. Exhale completely through your mouth for a count of eight. Repeat this cycle four times throughout the day, especially before meals.

Create Sacred Meal Space: Share meals with those who nourish your spirit. Engage in conversation that uplifts rather than depletes. Create physical environments that signal peace and presence—perhaps a beautiful place-mat, a single flower, or simply a cleared space without digital devices.

Positive Food Affirmations: As you prepare and enjoy your meals, practice affirmations that support relaxation such as "This food nourishes my entire being." "I trust my body's wisdom." "I am worthy of this nourishment." "My body knows how to receive what it needs from this meal."

Pleasure Practices: Explore activities that activate the same pleasure centers as comfort eating: movement that brings joy, creative expression, connection with nature, nurturing/intimate touch, or meditation. Notice when you're craving food but your body isn't physically hungry. This awareness creates space to choose alternative forms of nourishment.

Pre-Meal Ritual: Before eating, take three deep breaths. Place one hand on your heart and one on your belly. Acknowledge whatever emotions are present without judgment. Set an intention for how you wish to experience this meal. This simple thirty-second practice can dramatically shift your digestive capacity and your experience of nourishment.

Remember that healing your relationship with food is a pathway to healing your relationship with life itself. As you learn to relax into nourishment, you're simultaneously learning to embrace the fullness of your being—body, mind, heart, and spirit. This integration creates not just physical health but wholeness, the foundation for the vibrant midlife you deserve.

Chapter Summary

This chapter explores the intricate connections between our stress responses, gut health, hormonal balance, and eating patterns, particularly during midlife transitions. I explained how chronic stress triggers a cascade of physiological changes that affect digestion, nutrient absorption, and weight regulation. You also learned the concept of the enteric nervous system—our "second brain"—and the crucial role of the gut microbiome in overall health.

The chapter highlights how midlife hormonal shifts intensify these connections, creating new challenges that require understanding rather than self-blame. I offer practical approaches for cultivating a healthy gut-brain connection, reducing stress around meals, and creating a physiological state that supports natural appetite regulation and food freedom.

Personal Reflection Exercises

Exercise 1: Mapping Your Stress Response

Take a few moments to reflect on how stress manifests in your body and affects your eating patterns:

- When you feel stressed, where do you first notice it in your body? (Tension in shoulders, racing heart, stomach discomfort, etc.)

- What foods do you typically crave when under stress?

- How does your eating pace change when stressed?

- What digestion changes do you notice during stressful periods?

- How do you typically eat when stressed? (Standing, distracted, quickly, etc.)

On a blank page, draw an outline of a human body. Mark the areas where you personally experience stress sensations with one color. With another color, mark the areas where you notice changes in digestion or appetite regulation when stressed. Notice any patterns or connections between these marked areas.

Exercise 2: Your Nervous System States and Eating

The chapter discusses how our nervous system state—sympathetic (fight or flight) or parasympathetic (rest and digest)—profoundly affects our digestion and relationship with food.

For one week, before each meal, take a moment to assess your nervous system state:

- Rate your stress level from 1-10 (1 being completely relaxed, 10 being highly stressed)

- Note what you're doing while eating (working, watching TV, sitting at table, etc.)

- Observe how hungry you feel before eating (1-10 scale)

- After eating, note how satisfied you feel (1-10 scale)

- Record any digestive symptoms that follow

Look for patterns between your stress state during meals and your digestion, satisfaction, and hunger awareness. What insights emerge about your body's signals in different nervous system states?

Exercise 3: Midlife Hormonal Awareness Inventory

For women in midlife, hormonal shifts create new patterns in hunger, digestion, energy, and body composition. Take inventory of changes you've noticed in recent years:

Physical Changes:

- Hunger patterns and food cravings

- Digestive comfort or discomfort with foods previously well-tolerated

- Energy levels throughout the day

- Sleep quality and patterns

- Body composition and weight distribution

- Temperature regulation

- Skin changes

- Joint comfort

Emotional/Mental Changes:

- Mood stability

- Stress resilience

- Emotional relationship with food

- Food or body thoughts

- Memory and concentration

For each item where you've noticed significant change, ask your-self: "How have I been responding to this change? Have I been fighting against it or working with it? What might my body be asking for through this change?"

Exercise 4: Your Microbiome Support Assessment

The health of your gut microbiome affects not just digestion but also mood, immune function, and hormonal balance. Assess your current microbiome support:

Rate your intake of the following from 1-5 (1 = rarely/never, 5 = daily/abundant):

- Diverse plant foods (aim for 30+ different plant foods weekly)

- Fermented foods (yogurt, kefir, sauerkraut, kimchi, etc.)

- Prebiotic-rich foods (garlic, onions, asparagus, bananas, etc.)

- Colorful fruits and vegetables

- Adequate hydration

- Fiber-rich foods

Rate these factors from 1-5 (1 = significant concern, 5 = optimal):

- Stress management

- Sleep quality

- Regular movement

- Connection with nature

- Limited exposure to unnecessary antibiotics

- Minimally processed foods and artificial sweeteners

- Time for relaxed eating

Circle the three areas where improvement would be most beneficial for your gut health. What small, sustainable changes could you implement this week?

Journal Prompts

1. **Stress-Food Connection:** Reflect on the statement "your relationship with food often mirrors your more profound relationship with yourself and your life experiences." How do you see this connection playing out in your own life? When and how did you first notice the relationship between your stress levels and your eating patterns?

2. **Second Brain Wisdom:** The enteric nervous system (your second brain) communicates constantly with your central nervous system. What messages might your gut be sending that you've been overlooking? When have you experienced "gut feelings" that proved accurate in retrospect?

3. **Midlife Metabolic Adaptations:** Metabolic changes in midlife "aren't signs that your body is betraying you—they're adaptations requiring a more nuanced approach to nourishment and self-care." How might viewing these changes as adaptations rather than failures shift your relationship with your changing body? What would a more nuanced approach look like in your daily life?

4. **The French Paradox:** Consider the elements of traditional French eating habits described in the chapter (presence, pleasure, social connection, quality over quantity, etc.). Which of these elements feels most missing from your current relationship with food? Which one might be easiest to incorporate into your life now?

5. **Relaxation Response:** Recall a time when you ate in a truly relaxed state—perhaps on vacation, at a special celebration, or simply a moment when you were fully present with your food. How did this experience differ from your typical meals? How did your body respond?

Practice: Creating a Parasympathetic Eating Environment

This week, experiment with creating conditions that support your body's rest-and-digest mode during meals:

For One Meal Each Day:

1. **Prepare Your Space**

   - Clear your eating area of distractions (work materials, devices, clutter)

   - Add one element that signals "peaceful meal" to your nervous system (a candle, flowers, special placemat, beautiful dish)

   - Silence phone notifications or place your phone in another room

2. **Prepare Your Body**

   - Before eating, take three deep breaths (4-count inhale, 7-count hold, 8-count exhale)

   - Roll your shoulders gently up, back, and down

   - Place one hand on your heart and one on your belly for a moment

   - Say a brief statement of gratitude or set an intention

for this meal

3. During Your Meal

- Eat sitting down

- Take a moment to notice colors, aromas, and textures before beginning

- Put your utensils down between bites

- Chew thoroughly before swallowing

- Check in with your body midway through the meal. How does it feel?

4. After Your Meal

- Take a moment to notice how you feel physically and emotionally

- Give yourself 5-10 minutes before rushing to the next activity

- Note any differences in digestion, satisfaction, or energy compared to hurried meals

In your journal, record your observations: How did creating a parasympathetic-supportive environment change your eating experience? What was challenging about this practice? What was surprisingly easy or enjoyable?

Gut-Supporting Recipe Exercise

Experiment with creating a meal that incorporates multiple gut-supporting elements discussed in the chapter:

Design a meal that includes*:

- At least one fermented food

- At least one prebiotic-rich food

- A diversity of plant colors (aim for 3+ different colors)

- Adequate protein for midlife nutritional needs

- Healthy fats for hormone support

- Fiber for microbiome health

As you prepare and eat this meal:

- Notice the sensory experience of working with these foods

- Eat mindfully, considering the journey these foods will take through your digestive system

- After eating, note any observations about satisfaction, digestion, energy, and mood

Optional Extension: Invite friends or family to share this gut-supporting meal and discuss the mind-body-gut connection concepts from this chapter. How might shared knowledge about these connections transform your collective relationship with food?

*Please note: If you are under the care of a gastroenterologist and/or gut health coach, please confer with your team before embarking on adding any of these foods.

Stress-Response Awareness Practice

For moments when you feel the pull toward stress eating:

1. **Recognize the Urge:** Notice the physical sensations that signal stress or emotional eating urges (tension, racing heart, knot in stomach, etc.)

2. **Pause and Breathe:** Take three deep breaths to create space between the urge and your response

3. **Check In with Your Body:** Ask yourself:

   ○ "Am I physically hungry right now?"

   ○ "What emotion am I feeling at this moment?"

   ○ "What is my body truly needing?"

4. **Respond with Compassion:** Choose a response that addresses your actual need:

   ○ If physically hungry: Eat mindfully in a relaxed setting

- If emotionally activated but not hungry: Choose from a list of non-food soothing activities you've prepared in advance (short walk, cup of tea, stretching, journal for 3 minutes, call a friend, etc.)

- If unsure: Give yourself permission to wait 5-10 minutes while doing something nurturing, then reassess

5. **Release Judgment:** Whatever choice you make, practice self-compassion rather than criticism

Record instances when you practiced this awareness in your journal, noting what you discovered about your body's signals and needs.

Looking Forward

As you continue reading *Midlife Metamorphosis*, consider how the physiological understanding of the mind-body-gut connection provides a foundation for compassionate self-care. Notice how this knowledge might transform not just what you eat, but how you eat, and most importantly, how you relate to your body's wisdom during this significant life transition.

"Healing your relationship with food means honoring the wisdom of your body rather than fighting against it." - Mindy

The Mindful Path to Radical Acceptance

From Control to Freedom: A Personal Journey

I remember the afternoon and evening that illustrate my path toward healing, preparing pasta for my family during my restricting days. As I arranged ingredients, I noticed the serving size on the box: two ounces. I got out my food scale and measured thirty pieces of penne. I decided to allow myself just fifteen. While we gathered at the table, appearing to share a moment of connection, I was trapped in a mental prison, counting each piece that passed my lips. What should have been nourishment became another missed opportunity to connect with my loved ones, another moment where what I tried to control was controlling me.

This moment reflects a pattern many women recognize—the exhausting cycle of monitoring, restricting, and second-guessing our every choice. In those spaces between genuine living and constant vigilance, we lose not just pleasure but presence itself.

The Midlife Invitation to Awaken

As women approach midlife, we find ourselves at a pivotal juncture. Behind us lie decades of absorbing messages about how our bodies should look, what we should eat, and how much space we're allowed to occupy. Ahead lies the opportunity to reclaim what may have been lost—our innate wisdom, our sensory pleasure, and our rightful place at life's abundant table.

Midlife offers a unique neurological opportunity for transformation. Research indicates that the female brain undergoes remarkable changes during this transition. Dr. Christiane Northrup, a women's health pioneer, describes how fluctuating hormones during perimenopause and menopause can disrupt established neural pathways, initially causing distress but ultimately creating space for new neural connections. This neuroplasticity presents a biological window for profound change, allowing us to shed conditioning that no longer serves us and embrace new ways of being.[1]

This is why many women report a growing sense of authenticity, courage, and self-acceptance as they move through midlife. What some call a "crisis" is actually a powerful invitation to awaken.

---

1. Northrup, Christiane. The Wisdom of Menopause: Creating Physical and Emotional Health During the Change. Revised and Updated. Bantam Books, 2012, pp. 97-103.

Clearing the Clutter

We all know the feeling of overwhelm. Our days overflow with responsibilities—errands, emails, work demands, and relationships. These endless to-do lists can create the sensation that time is slipping through our fingers. We find ourselves eating on the run, eating in the car, eating in front of screens, multitasking, or standing absent-mindedly at the refrigerator. In these moments, pleasure and calm become distant memories. The time has come to clear this clutter from our eating experience.

The pace of modern life affects women disproportionately. Research from the American Psychological Association shows that women consistently report higher stress levels than men, with midlife women often carrying the heaviest load such as balancing careers, family responsibilities, aging parents, and their own changing health needs.[2] This stress directly impacts our relationship with food, as cortisol elevations trigger cravings and disrupt our natural hunger and satiety signals.

When we embrace mindful eating, free from distraction, we rediscover the art of savoring and appreciating our food. Eating transforms into a sensory celebration. Pleasure becomes the cornerstone of food freedom. In pleasure's presence, guilt, shame, and fear cannot survive.

---

2. American Psychological Association. (2020). Stress in America™ 2020: A National Mental Health Crisis.

Mindful eating invites us to discover and delight in the sight, aroma, texture, and flavor of our food. By honoring the moment and slowing down, we fully experience every element, raising awareness that naturally guides us toward satisfying portions.

Eating with both mindfulness and soul connection allows us to cultivate a relationship with food that is not just healthy but truly freeing.

The Wisdom of Mindfulness: Ancient Practice Meets Modern Science

Mindfulness has roots in ancient Buddhist meditation practices dating back over two-thousand-plus years. Its essence is raising heightened awareness of our behaviors, thoughts, and emotions without judgment. While these practices emerged from spiritual traditions, modern neuroscience confirms their transformative power.

Dr. Jon Kabat-Zinn, founder of Mindfulness-Based Stress Reduction (MBSR), brought these practices into Western medicine in the 1970s. [3] Since then, thousands of studies have documented mindfulness's effects on the brain and body. Particularly relevant

---

3. Kabat-Zinn, Jon. *Full Catastrophe Living: Using the Wisdom of Your Body and Mind to Face Stress, Pain, and Illness.* Revised and Updated Edition. Bantam Books, 2013, pp.3-2 0. https://www.apa.org/news/press/releases/stress/2020/sia -mental-health-crisis.pdf

for women in midlife is research showing that regular mindfulness practice can reduce the intensity of hot flashes, improve sleep quality, and decrease anxiety—all common challenges during this life phase. Mindful eating isn't about obsessing over food choices or counting calories. It's about becoming exquisitely aware of your body's signals whenever you eat. Through mindful eating, you begin to observe the subtle cues that influence how, what, and when you nourish yourself.

The Body's Wisdom: How Mindfulness Transforms Digestion

Eating with awareness holds profound power. It creates space to honor your hunger and recognize satisfaction. It activates the relaxation response that enhances digestion and nutrient absorption and supports every system in your magnificent body.

This process begins in your mind. Scientists call it the Cephalic Phase Digestive Response (CPDR)—cephalic meaning "of the head." This digestive phase encompasses the pleasures of taste, smell, satisfaction, and the visual delight of a meal. It's about how our minds participate in digestion. Research suggests that thirty to forty percent of our digestive response to any meal comes from this mental awareness.

Digestion awakens in the mind as receptors on your tongue, in your mouth, and nose respond to smelling, tasting, chewing, and simply noticing your food. True awareness of your meal initiates saliva production, stomach acid, enzymes, neuropeptides, and the full spectrum of pancreatic enzymes. Simultaneously, blood flows to your digestive organs, your stomach and intestines begin their rhythmic dance, and electrolytes prepare to welcome nourishment.

When we eat without awareness, not registering taste, smell, satisfaction, or visual elements, we digest and metabolize at only sixty to seventy percent capacity. This results in less efficient digestion, nutrient absorption, and metabolism.

A fascinating study on "dichotomous listening" illustrates this connection. Participants listened to two people speaking simultaneously, one in the left ear discussing space travel, the other in the right ear talking about financial freedom. When relaxed, these participants absorbed minerals at one-hundred percent efficiency. When exposed to divided attention and given the same mineral drink, they showed minimal absorption. The simple act of dividing attention dramatically affected digestive metabolism. [4]

For midlife women, this science is particularly relevant. Many experience digestive changes during perimenopause and menopause, including increased bloating, constipation, reflux,

---

4. David, Marc. *Nourishing Wisdom: A Mind-Body Approach to Nutrition and Well-Being.* Bell Tower, 1991, pp. 76-79.

and food sensitivities. Mindful eating can help manage these symptoms by optimizing the digestive process from its very beginning.

When our awareness drifts outside our bodies, we cannot experience the physical sensations connected with food. We miss the signals of fullness, the pleasure of flavors, or even our true preferences.

When we question our food choices, focusing on what we believe is "bad" or whether we should be eating it at all, mindfulness becomes impossible. Like conversing with a distracted friend, we leave the table feeling incomplete and wanting more.

The cephalic phase is actually a nutritional requirement. Your brain must experience taste, pleasure, aroma, and satisfaction to initiate efficient digestion. When eating hastily or without attention, your brain interprets this as hunger, prompting you to eat more. The less awareness disappears at the table, the more you need to consume. When eating amid distractions, flavor disappears, and your brain signals, "I want more."

The same phenomenon occurs when guilt, shame, and fear cloud your food choices. That donut, chocolate, or pasta goes unnoticed. What you thought you wanted brings no satisfaction. How can we empower ourselves with confident choices when we don't fully allow ourselves to have them?

Breaking the Cycle: Midlife as Opportunity

What makes midlife such a powerful time to transform our relationship with food? Beyond the neuroplasticity mentioned earlier, this life stage brings several advantages:

First, we must embrace the wisdom of experience. By midlife, many women have tried numerous diets and restrictive eating patterns, only to find themselves caught in cycles of deprivation and overeating. This lived experience creates readiness for a new approach.

Second, midlife often brings a deeper understanding of life's preciousness and brevity. As we become more aware of time's passage, many women feel a growing urgency to live authentically and joyfully. The question shifts from "How do I look?" to "How do I want to live?"

Third, research shows that women's focus often shifts from external validation to internal satisfaction around midlife. Dr. Mary Pipher, in her groundbreaking work on women's development, notes that this natural evolution toward authenticity creates fertile ground for practices like mindful eating, which prioritize internal wisdom over external rules. [5]

---

5. Pipher, Mary. *Women Rowing North: Navigating Life's Currents and Flourishing As We Age*. Bloomsbury Publishing, 2019.

Many women share that midlife brought a sudden realization: "I've spent thirty years at war with my body. How much longer will I continue this battle?" This recognition can spark a revolutionary shift toward peace and acceptance.

Embodied Wisdom: The Path to Radical Acceptance

One powerful strategy for developing a healthy relationship with food through mindfulness is embodiment. Embodiment means fully inhabiting your body, honoring, and respecting the space where you feel relaxed and empowered. In this space, pleasure flourishes. Here, you experience the heightened physical sensations of eating without guilt or shame.

Dr. Bessel van der Kolk, trauma researcher and author of *The Body Keeps the Score*, [6] explains that many women become disconnected from their bodies due to cultural messaging, past trauma, or chronic stress. Mindfulness practices gently restore this connection, allowing us to reclaim our physical selves as safe, trustworthy homes.

Embodiment doesn't mean obsessing over every bodily sensation. Rather, it means developing a compassionate awareness of your body's signals and honoring them with respect. This practice is particularly powerful in midlife, when many women feel betrayed by bodies that seem to be changing beyond their control.

---

6. van der Kolk, Bessel A. *The Body Keeps the Score: Brain, Mind, and Body in the Healing of Trauma*. Penguin Books, 2014.

Practicing mindfulness and embodiment keeps you present rather than using food to disconnect. Embodiment reflects your body's innate wisdom and how attuned you are to it. Eating what you want and need, when you want and need it, becomes possible only when you include your body in the conversation. Relying on external measures like scales, distorted self-images, or someone else's rules disconnects you from mindfulness and embodiment.

> **The mindful eater naturally checks in with her body for fullness cues. Even while multitasking, she remains connected to her body's messages because the signals are clear and trustworthy.**

Mindful eaters breathe during meals, chew thoroughly, pause often to savor flavors, and focus on the present meal rather than dwelling on past choices or future plans.

The Neuroscience of Self-Compassion

Central to radical acceptance is self-compassion by treating ourselves with the same kindness we would offer a dear friend. For many midlife women, self-compassion feels foreign after decades of harsh self-criticism.

Neuroscience helps explain why self-compassion transforms our relationship with food. Dr. Kelly McGonigal's research shows that self-criticism activates the brain's threat cravings. [7] Conversely, self-compassion activates the care-giving system, releasing oxytocin and creating feelings of safety and contentment.

This biological understanding helps explain why punitive approaches to eating, like strict diets or self-criticism after indulgences, ultimately backfire. They activate our stress response, making mindful choices nearly impossible.

Dr. Kristin Neff identifies three components of self-compassion that can transform our relationship with food:[8]

1. Mindfulness: Observing our thoughts and feelings without judgment

2. Common humanity: Recognizing that struggle is part of the shared human experience

3. Self-kindness: Treating ourselves with care and understanding

When we bring these elements to our eating experience, radical acceptance becomes possible. We can acknowledge our humanity—our cravings, our pleasure in food, our occasional overindul-

---

7. McGonigal, Kelly. *The Willpower Instinct: How Self-Control Works, Why It Matters, and What You Can Do to Get More of It*. Avery, 2012, pp. 145-148.

8. Neff, Kristin. *Self-Compassion: The Proven Power of Being Kind to Yourself*. William Morrow, 2011, pp. 41-44.

gence—without harsh judgment. This acceptance, paradoxically, creates the safety needed for lasting change.

Mindful eating opens the door to unprecedented freedom. Trusting your body's natural intelligence empowers you to embrace the delicious gifts food offers. Mindful eating invites not just a healthy relationship with food, but a loving one.

From Compulsion to Compassion

Let me be clear: A compulsive eater is not a food lover. Craving, obsessing, bingeing, and restricting do not reflect love. Eating from fear, guilt, or the need to escape reflects lost connection sparked by negative self-talk and shame.

Compulsive eating robs you of food's pleasures because you fear what it will do *to* you while believing you're not permitted to enjoy it. You might eat "acceptable" foods while finding covert ways to consume what you truly desire, distracting yourself from your eating reality.

Research on the neurobiology of compulsive eating reveals that restriction actually primes the brain for bingeing. Dr. Ancel Keys' famous Minnesota Starvation Experiment demonstrates that even mentally healthy individuals developed food obsessions, bingeing behaviors, and emotional distress when subjected to restriction. For midlife women who have spent decades cycling through diets, this research validates their experience: The problem wasn't lack of willpower, but rather a natural biological response to perceived scarcity.[9]

Regardless of your weight, you deserve pleasure and joy in your food, just as you deserve pleasure and joy in all aspects of life. This isn't indulgence; it's your birthright.

Loving food means engaging all senses, smelling, tasting, savoring. A love affair with food gives new meaning to emotional eating. Yes, you read correctly—emotional eating can be wonderful. Eating WITH emotion rather than eating TO manage emotions is transformative. When you eat, fully experience the wonder and complexity of food as you embrace freedom.

The Practice of Radical Acceptance

Radical acceptance means embracing reality completely, with compassion and without resistance. Applied to our bodies and food, it means acknowledging our hunger, our pleasure, and our physical form, exactly as they are in this moment. Not as we wish they were. Not as society tells us they should be. But as they authentically are.

This doesn't mean passive resignation. Rather, you can create the foundation for meaningful change. Only when we fully ac-

---

9. Keys, Ancel, Josef Brožek, Austin Henschel, Olaf Mickelsen, and Henry Longstreet Taylor. *The Biology of Human Starvation* (2 volumes). University of Minnesota Press, 1950.

knowledge where we are can we move intentionally toward where we want to be.

For midlife women, radical acceptance might include:

- Acknowledging the natural changes in metabolism and body composition that accompany aging

- Honoring hunger as a legitimate biological signal, not an enemy to be conquered

- Recognizing pleasure as essential to well-being, not an indulgence to be earned

- Accepting that healing one's relationship with food is a practice, not a perfect performance

- Embracing the wisdom that comes with lived experience in a society that often devalues aging women

Dr. Tara Brach, psychologist and author of *Radical Acceptance*, describes this practice as "clearly recognizing what is happening inside us and regarding what we see with an open, kind, and loving heart." This clarity and kindness create the conditions for transf ormation.[10]

---

10. Brach, Tara. Radical Acceptance: Embracing Your Life with the Heart of a Buddha. Bantam Books, 2004.

A Taste of Freedom: My Personal Journey

Years ago, I discovered a vegetarian chili recipe—a PLEASURE food for me. I kept the recipe tucked away until finally preparing it on a cold winter evening. After gathering ingredients, I tasted, seasoned, tasted again, simmered, stirred, and savored once more. The result delighted me.

Why share this seemingly ordinary story?

Not long ago, after spending most of my adult life restricting, eating compulsively, and purging, I recognized that my obsession with food, dieting, and my body had finally lifted. That soul-warming pot of chili represented my transformation. Gone were the mental calculations of calories, fat, protein, and carbs. Instead, I focused on taste, texture, and the pure deliciousness of my meal. As my senses awakened, so did my sense of self. I realized I no longer needed to be the smallest person in the room or judge myself by the size of my body. I developed a sense of self that inspired me to expand—in spirit—to claim more space on this blessed earth. I no longer feared what food would do TO me and fully embraced what it could do FOR me. I'm happy to share this recipe with you (see the end of this chapter) and hope that you find it to be as delicious as I do, on many levels.

My journey reflects a truth that researchers are increasingly confirming: Lasting peace with food comes not through greater control but through greater acceptance. A 2020 review in the International Journal of Eating Disorders examining intuitive eating (which incorporates mindfulness principles) found that this approach was associated with improved psychological health, better body image, and healthier physiological markers—without the weight cycling and psychological distress that often accompany restrictive diets. [11]

Creating Your Mindful Midlife

The journey to acceptance through mindfulness isn't a straight path. It's a spiral, returning us again and again to the same lessons with deeper understanding each time. Here are practices that can support your journey:

1. **Begin with compassionate awareness**: Before changing anything, simply notice your current patterns around food with kindness. What triggers automatic eating? When do you feel most connected to your body's signals? When do you feel disconnected?

2. **Create mindful eating spaces**: Designate at least one meal daily as a mindfulness practice. Remove distractions, set a beautiful table (even just for yourself), and bring full attention to the sensory experience.

---

11. Linardon, J., Tylka, T. L., & Fuller-Tyszkiewicz, M. (2021). Intuitive eating and its psychological correlates: A meta-analysis. International Journal of Eating Disorders, 54(7), 1149-1170. https://doi.org/10.1002/eat.23509

3. **Develop a gratitude practice**: Before meals, take a moment to appreciate the nourishment before you, the hands that grew and prepared it, the earth that sustained it, the body that will receive it.

4. **Cultivate community**: Share your journey with like-minded women. Research shows that social support significantly enhances our ability to maintain positive changes.

5. **Be gentle with yourself**: Remember that mindfulness is a practice, not a performance. Each meal offers a new opportunity to begin again.

The midlife journey toward radical acceptance (your fully nourished life) isn't about achieving perfection. It's about reclaiming the wisdom and pleasure that have always been yours. It's about recognizing that the path to peace with food lies not in stricter control but in deeper connection—with your body, your authentic needs, and the sensory pleasures that make life worth savoring.

The next time you reach for comfort food, consider what will truly bring peace and pleasure to your soul. Eat it with awareness and without guilt, and welcome all the healing and nourishment it offers you. This, my friend, is your birthright, not just in midlife, but in every precious moment of your journey.

Chapter Summary

In this transformative chapter, I explored how mindfulness creates the foundation for radical acceptance and food freedom. I shared my personal journey from counting pasta pieces to fully enjoying a soul-warming vegetarian chili, illustrating how midlife offers a unique opportunity for awakening and transformation. The chapter explains the science behind mindful eating, including the cephalic phase digestive response that accounts for thirty to forty percent of our digestive efficiency, and how reconnecting with our bodies' wisdom through embodiment practices leads to greater peace with food.

I distinguished between compulsive eating and truly loving food, emphasizing that eating WITH emotion (fully present and engaged) differs profoundly from eating TO manage emotions. I introduced the neuroscience of self-compassion and how it creates the conditions for healing our relationship with food. The chapter culminates in an understanding that radical acceptance—embracing reality exactly as it is without resistance—creates the foundation for meaningful change in our relationship with food and our bodies.

Recipe: Who Woulda Thunk It Chili

(Adapted from Clean and Delicious). For more great recipes, visit https://the-freedom-promise.kit.com/recipes. Makes 10 cups.

Ingredients

1 large onion, chopped

4 cloves garlic, peeled and crushed

2 bell peppers, 1 red and 1 green, seeded and chopped into 1-inch pieces

¼-½ jalapeno pepper, seeded and diced, to taste

4 cups of butternut squash, cut into 1-inch pieces**

4 - 15 oz. cans of beans, rinsed and drained (I used 2 cans of red kidney, 1 can of black beans and 1 can of pinto beans)

½ bunch cilantro, chopped

2 Tbsp. chili powder

1 Tbsp. cumin

1 - 15 oz. can fire roasted tomatoes

4 cups low sodium vegetable broth

½ bunch kale, stemmed and chopped

1 Tbsp. extra virgin olive oil

Salt and freshly ground pepper, to taste

Directions

Heat olive oil in a large pot over medium heat. Once heated, add onions, garlic and jalapeno, with a small pinch of salt. Cook for about 2 minutes, stirring occasionally.

Stir in bell peppers and cook for another 2 minutes. Add squash, chili powder, cumin and stir well. Add beans, tomatoes and broth. Turn heat to high and bring to a boil. Once boiling, reduce to a simmer and cook until the squash is tender, about 45 minutes. Continue simmering until the chili reaches your desired consistency; the longer it simmers, the thicker the chili.

Add the kale to the pot and cover for about 5 minutes or until it wilts down. Give everything one last stir...taste it...adjust the seasoning. Finish with the chopped cilantro.

I served this chili with accompaniments of guacamole and gluten free tortilla chips. Delish!

Personal Reflection Exercises

Exercise 1: Uncovering Your Mindfulness Barriers

Consider the factors that most frequently pull you away from present-moment awareness during meals:

Create a personal "mindfulness barriers" inventory by rating how frequently these common distractions affect your eating experience (1 = rarely, 5 = nearly always):

- Electronic devices (phones, television, computers)

- Reading material (books, magazines, mail)

- Work-related activities or thoughts

- Family responsibilities or interruptions

- Worry about past or future meals/choices

- Critical thoughts about your food or body

- Rush/time pressure

- Emotional distress

- Environmental distractions (noise, uncomfortable setting)

- Other: _____

For your three highest-rated barriers, reflect:

- When did this pattern begin?

- What need is it attempting to meet?

- What small step could you take to reduce this barrier's impact?

Exercise 2: The Cephalic Phase Experience

This exercise helps you experience firsthand the power of the cephalic phase digestive response discussed in the chapter:

Part 1: Mindless Eating - Choose a small portion of food you enjoy. Before beginning, set a timer for 2 minutes.

- Eat while engaging in a distracting activity (scrolling on your phone, watching TV, reading)

- Try to finish the portion before the timer ends

- Immediately after, note:

  - How much flavor you experienced

  - Your level of satisfaction

  - Any physical sensations you notice

  - Whether you could accurately describe what you just ate

Part 2: Mindful Eating (at least 1 hour later) - Choose the same food in the same portion. Set your timer for 2 minutes again.

- Eliminate all distractions

- Before eating, notice the appearance, aroma, and texture

- Eat slowly, savoring each bite fully

- Notice the flavors, textures, and your body's responses

- Stop when the timer rings, whether you've finished or not

Reflection Questions:

- How did your experience of the same food differ between the two approaches?

- How did your satisfaction level compare?

- What physical differences did you notice in your digestive response?

- What does this experiment reveal about the role of awareness in your eating experience?

Exercise 3: Body Wisdom Mapping

This exercise helps reconnect you with your body's inherent wisdom:

On a blank page, draw a simple outline of a human body. Using different colors, mark the areas where you experience these various sensations:

- Physical hunger (empty stomach, growling, energy dip, etc.)

- Satisfaction/fullness

- Pleasure in eating

- Stress or tension during meals

- Connection to emotional eating patterns

- Places that hold judgment or shame

- Areas of appreciation and gratitude

After completing your map, reflect:

- Which sensations are easiest for you to identify?

- Which are most challenging to recognize?

- Where do you notice disconnection from your body's signals?

- What patterns emerge when you view these sensations visually?

Keep this map accessible and update it periodically as you develop greater bodily awareness. Notice how the map evolves as you practice mindful eating.

Exercise 4: Radical Acceptance Practice

Radical acceptance is described as "embracing reality completely, without resistance." This exercise helps you explore what radical acceptance might mean for your relationship with food and body:

Part 1: Current Reality Write honest, non-judgmental responses to these prompts:

- The current reality of my body is...

- The current reality of my relationship with food is...

- The current reality of my thoughts about eating is...

- The current reality of my feelings during meals is...

Part 2: Resistance Patterns For each reality you described, identify how you typically resist this truth:

- I resist the reality of my body by...

- I resist the reality of my relationship with food by...

- I resist the reality of my thoughts about eating by...

- I resist the reality of my feelings during meals by...

Part 3: Acceptance Exploration Now, imagine what full acceptance might feel like:

- If I fully accepted the reality of my body, I might...

- If I fully accepted the reality of my relationship with food, I might...

- If I fully accepted the reality of my thoughts about eating, I might...

- If I fully accepted the reality of my feelings during meals, I might...

Remember that acceptance doesn't mean resignation or giving up on change. Rather, it creates the foundation from which meaningful transformation can emerge.

Journal Prompts

1. **Midlife Awakening:** I described midlife as "a powerful intersection" and "a biological window for profound change." How has your relationship with food and body shifted as you've entered or moved through midlife? What aspects of yourself are awakening or seeking expression at this life stage?

2. **Mental Clutter:** The chapter discusses how clearing the clutter from our eating experience creates space for pleasure and presence. What mental clutter most commonly

accompanies your meals? How might your eating experience transform if you could release this mental noise?

3. **Embodiment Exploration:** Reflect on the statement that "embodiment means fully inhabiting your body, honoring and respecting the space where you feel relaxed and empowered." When do you feel most embodied and present in your physical self? What activities, environments, or practices help you reconnect with your body's wisdom?

4. **Self-Compassion Practice:** Dr. Kristin Neff identifies three components of self-compassion: mindfulness, common humanity, and self-kindness. Which of these elements comes most naturally to you, and which feels most challenging? How might developing greater self-compassion transform your relationship with food?

5. **From Control to Freedom:** I shared my personal journey from counting pasta pieces to fully enjoying a nourishing vegetarian chili. What would true food freedom look like in your life? What specific beliefs or behaviors would you release, and what new experiences might become possible?

Practice: The Mindful Meal Experience

This week, commit to at least three fully mindful meals, following this practice:

Before the Meal:

1. **Create Sacred Space:**

   - Remove distractions (phones, television, reading materials)

   - Set an intentional eating environment (perhaps a place-mat, a candle, or a flower)

   - Take three deep breaths to center yourself

2. **Express Gratitude:**

   - Acknowledge the sources of your food

   - Appreciate your body's ability to receive nourishment

   - Note one aspect of the meal you're looking forward to experiencing

During the Meal:

1. **Engage Your Senses:**

   - Notice colors, aromas, textures before taking the first

bite

- ○ Chew thoroughly, exploring the flavors fully

- ○ Place your utensils down between bites

2. **Body Awareness:**

- ○ Check in with your body midway through the meal

- ○ Notice sensations of satisfaction emerging

- ○ Pause if you notice yourself rushing

After the Meal:
1. **Reflective Integration:**

- ○ Note your level of satisfaction without judgment

- ○ Observe your energy and mood

- ○ Express gratitude for the nourishment received

Reflection Journal: After each mindful meal, briefly record:

- What you noticed about the sensory experience

- How your digestion felt compared to less mindful meals

- What emotions or thoughts arose during the practice

- One insight you gained from this experience

By the end of the week, review your reflections and note any patterns or changes in your eating experience as your mindfulness practice develops.

Self-Compassion Break for Food-Related Stress

This practice, adapted from Dr. Kristin Neff's work, provides a way to respond with kindness when food-related stress or judgment arises:

When you notice yourself experiencing food-related stress, judgment, or anxiety:

1. **Mindfulness:** Place your hand on your heart and acknowledge your experience:

   - "This is a moment of suffering" or "This is challenging"

   - "I'm noticing judgment/anxiety/shame about food right now"

2. **Common Humanity:** Recognize your shared experience with others:

   - "I'm not alone in this struggle"

   - "Many women have faced similar challenges with food and body"

   - "This is part of being human in our culture"

3. **Self-Kindness:** Offer yourself compassion:

   ○ "May I be kind to myself in this moment"

   ○ "May I give myself the compassion I need"

   ○ "I'm doing the best I can with the resources I have right now"

4. **Supportive Touch:** Maintain your hand on your heart, or move your hand to any part of your body that needs comfort

5. **Deep Breath:** Take a full, centering breath before continuing with your day

This practice takes just 30-60 seconds and can be done anywhere—before meals, while grocery shopping, when trying on clothes, or whenever food-related stress arises. With practice, it becomes a powerful tool for interrupting self-criticism and creating space for mindful choices.

Embodiment Practice: The 5-Minute Body Reunion

This simple daily practice helps rebuild trust and connection with your body:

Find a quiet space where you won't be interrupted. Sit or lie down comfortably.

1. **Begin with Grounding:**

- Close your eyes or soften your gaze

- Feel the points of contact between your body and the surface supporting you

- Take three deep breaths, allowing your body to relax with each exhale

2. **Body Scan:**

- Bringing kind awareness to each area of your body, starting at your feet

- Notice sensations without judgment, temperature, pressure, tingling, etc.

- Acknowledge any areas of tension or discomfort with compassion

- Express gratitude for what each body part enables you to experience

3. **Wisdom Inquiry:**

- Ask your body: "What do you need from me today?"

- Listen patiently for any signals or messages that arise

- These might come as sensations, images, words, or simply knowing

4. **Integration:**

- Identify one small way you can honor your body's wisdom today

- This might be movement, rest, specific nourishment, or emotional release

- Set an intention to respond to this need with kindness

5. **Closure:**

- Place your hands over your heart in a gesture of care

- Thank your body for its constant support and wisdom

- Return to your day with this embodied awareness

Practice this body reunion daily, ideally at the same time (perhaps morning or evening), to rebuild trust with your body's signals and wisdom. Over time, you'll likely notice greater ease in recognizing hunger, fullness, and other bodily messages throughout your day.

Looking Forward

As you continue your journey through *Midlife Metamorphosis*, notice how mindfulness and radical acceptance create a foundation for the food freedom you're cultivating. When you bring present-moment awareness to your eating experience, you create space for pleasure, satisfaction, and true nourishment. This mindful presence builds upon the hunger awareness work from the previous chapter and prepares you for deeper exploration of other aspects of nourishment beyond food.

Remember that radical acceptance is both a destination and a continuing practice. Some days will flow more easily than others. What matters most is your willingness to return to presence with compassion rather than judgment, knowing that each meal offers a new opportunity to connect with your body's inherent wisdom.

"Loving food means engaging all senses—smelling, tasting, savoring. A love affair with food gives new meaning to emotional eating ...Eating WITH emotion rather than eating TO manage emotions is transformative." - Mindy

Honoring Your Hunger

The Path to Food Freedom

Understanding true physical hunger, emotional hunger and toxic hunger forms the foundation for developing a nourishing relationship with food and your body.

Physical Hunger: Your Body's Wisdom

Your body is an exquisite creation of evolutionary brilliance. The hunger regulation system that evolved over millions of years is a testament to your body's inherent wisdom—a delicate balance between fuel intake and energy expenditure. This ancient system of survival has kept humanity thriving through feast and famine.

At the center of this magnificent intelligence is your hypothalamus, which orchestrates a symphony of hormones to guide your eating patterns. When your body senses its energy reserves are low, it releases ghrelin—your hunger hormone—signaling that nourishment is needed. This isn't merely a physical sensation but a powerful evolutionary mechanism that ensured our ancestors sought food when resources were available.

Simultaneously, insulin works to regulate your blood sugar levels, while leptin—your satiety hormone—produces feelings of fullness and contentment, guiding you to stop eating when you've received adequate nourishment. This delicate hormonal dance evolved as a survival adaptation, ensuring humans consumed enough energy to thrive without depleting precious resources.

For many women who have lived through chronic dieting cycles, hunger becomes just another sensation to suppress. They've become remarkably efficient at ignoring these vital signals, disconnecting from their innate ability to trust their natural biological wisdom. In these cycles, it's easy to forget that food represents both nourishment and pleasure, it honors our complete humanity.

As infants, our first experiences of love and nurturing occurred as we were held and fed. Later, we may have developed beautiful associations with food through memories of a beloved grandmother's kitchen or cherished holiday traditions. These associations can transform into relationship patterns that shape how we respond to life's challenges. At some point, many of us discovered that coming home after a difficult day and indulging in cookies or chips provided temporary relief.

**The mind records this pattern: feel bad → eat →
feel better.**

The hunger signal becomes lost in this emotional translation. Each time we experience distress, our minds remember this reliable comfort strategy. We've learned to seek momentary pleasure to avoid immediate discomfort. This fleeting relief is chemical by nature, and the highly refined, sugar-rich foods most often sought create a powerful blood sugar response that generates sensations of pleasure and relaxation. When this response subsides, painful emotions return, we seek more comfort, and a self-perpetuating cycle emerges.

In my journey, when I refused to honor my body's hunger signals—essentially restricting myself throughout the day, dismissing any calls for nourishment—I unknowingly created the perfect conditions for episodes of evening overeating. I played mental games with myself: how few calories could I consume before dinner? Breakfast might have been a carefully measured portion of cereal with skim milk and perhaps a few berries. Mid-morning would bring more coffee to suppress hunger, and lunch would consist of a modest salad with fat-free dressing or perhaps a fat-free yogurt.

If I managed to endure the afternoon without surrendering to pantry temptations, finishing my children's after-school snacks, or sampling dinner preparations, by evening my body would be loudly announcing its desperation for nourishment. Dinner became my largest meal, and I typically ate well past fullness. After dinner, I would seek relief from the day's accumulated stress through something salty, sweet, creamy, or crunchy. I would fall asleep uncomfortably full, promising myself to "do better" tomorrow.

There is no benefit in silencing your body's wisdom. We must learn to include our physical selves in this sacred conversation because while our minds may remain tethered to toxic beliefs that certain foods will make us gain weight, eventually our bodies will assert their truth, reminding us they need proper nutrients to support brain function and hormonal balance. Eating when genuinely hungry—tuning into your body's signals for nourishment—dramatically improves the likelihood that you won't find yourself holding an empty container of ice cream after a day of trying to be "good."

When we restrict foods that bring us pleasure or act upon thoughts and beliefs that create nutritional deprivation, we inevitably crave what our bodies genuinely need for energy, including those foods we've deemed "forbidden," such as fats and carbohydrates. By not trusting our hunger, we create a landscape of deprivation, feelings of failure, and ultimately, powerlessness around food. I invite you to identify your cravings and listen to their wisdom. Hunger tells us when to eat; cravings guide us toward what to eat.

Eating when hungry and stopping when satisfied is more about HOW, WHY, and WHEN we eat than WHAT we eat. The WHAT continually evolves as nutrition science discovers new insights and establishes new rules and guidelines. The WHAT will evolve due to the changing needs of our bodies as we move through the seasons of life. These factors remain constant whether we're enjoying tofu or tacos.

There is profound empowerment in choosing your food wisely, eating in a gentle rhythm to savor and find satisfaction, relaxing into the experience to support digestion and nutrient absorption, and allowing your body to be energized as it receives these benefits.

Emotional Hunger: The Heart's Yearning

We eat emotionally, seeking comfort during highly charged circumstances. Often, our true desire isn't for the food itself but for the emotional state it temporarily creates.

Creating space between our behaviors and feelings is essential for transformation.

We frequently turn to food to distract ourselves from boredom and emotional discomfort. During my late husband Stuart's cancer treatments in the hospital, I spent countless hours alone while he slept or remained sedated from medications. Walking the halls inevitably led me to the cafeteria. Filling myself with bitter coffee, unsatisfying salads, mealy apples, stale bagels, and sugar-laden yogurts became a way to pass time. I wasn't experiencing physical hunger; I was bored, fearful, grieving, and lonely. More nourishing responses would have included calling a friend, writing in my journal, or visiting the chapel to acknowledge what I was genuinely feeling.

Occasionally we reach for food when what we truly need is human connection, a warm embrace, meaningful connection, genuine security, and authentic intimacy. These "cravings" emerge from parts of ourselves that may be yearning for love, connection, and fulfillment.

We often celebrate joyous occasions like job promotions with cupcakes and champagne. Food naturally accompanies life's celebrations, and we may overindulge because we're unaccustomed to receiving pleasure from food as a regular, guilt-free experience.

Several distinctions separate emotional hunger from physical hunger. I emphasize these distinctions because many women have lost touch with the difference, especially after years of denying their true hunger signals:

- Emotional hunger arrives suddenly and demands immediate satisfaction, while physical hunger develops gradually, allowing you time to respond mindfully.

- When eating to fill an emotional void, you typically crave specific comfort foods, such as pizza or ice cream. When responding to authentic physical hunger, you remain open to nourishing options.

- When eating in response to emotions or stress, you're likely to continue past fullness. When satisfying genuine hunger, you're more attuned to your body's signals of satisfaction and fullness.

Toxic Hunger: The Body's Protest

Toxic hunger refers to withdrawal symptoms that emerge from consuming foods with minimal nutritional value, better known as ultra-processed foods, which are essentially science experiments disguised as food. These symptoms occur when experiencing blood sugar crashes, driving our bodies to consume more than needed in response to intense cravings, contributing to weight fluctuations, and making sustainable weight management more challenging.

If you're reading this book, you've likely been consuming foods marketed as light, fat-free, and sugar-free—essentially disconnected from real nourishment. Common symptoms of toxic hunger include:
- Emptiness sensations in the stomach
- Stomach gurgling and rumbling
- Dizziness, lightheadedness, headaches
- Irritability and agitation
- Concentration difficulties
- Nausea, shakiness, and fatigue

True hunger, unlike toxic hunger, signals when your body requires calories to maintain energy levels and preserve lean body mass. When we eat in harmony with our body's innate wisdom, maintaining a healthy weight becomes natural. In our current food environment, many of us have lost our connection to this wisdom and the signals guiding us toward appropriate portions and genuinely nourishing foods. The path back from a relationship with food entangled in toxicity begins with examining our beliefs and patterns, questioning whether they serve our highest good, and making empowered choices toward transformation.

Cravings: Your Body's Messengers

Sometimes hunger manifests as cravings, and cravings often emerge in response to extreme hunger or nutritional imbalances.

Cravings represent your body's sophisticated communication system signaling that something is missing—a story about an underlying health concern or a biochemical and nutritional element you may need.

Often we crave sugar when our bodies actually need protein or rest. Salt cravings might indicate a need for essential minerals like potassium, chromium, or copper, suggesting you incorporate more mineral-rich foods like nuts, seeds, and sea vegetables. Chocolate cravings may signal an iron or magnesium requirement, pointing toward more leafy greens like kale or bok choy.

Occasionally, the message extends beyond nutrition into deeper realms of fulfillment. Are you hearing "I need chocolate" when you truly may seek spirituality, sensuality, movement, joy, or creative expression? That piece of cake might represent a desire for more sweetness in your life. Truthfully, reaching for candy is simpler than exploring the depths of what might lie beyond our comfort zones. The cravings triggered by emotional responses transcend food. When experiencing a craving, approach it with gentle curiosity and ask what may need balance.

Consider this mindful checklist the next time a craving emerges to discover what you're truly hungry for:

- When did you last nourish yourself?

- Did your previous meal or snack include sufficient protein, fat, and fiber? A proper choice would be avocado toast with an egg or full-fat (yes, full-fat) Greek yogurt with a handful of nuts and berries.

- How was the quality of your sleep last night? Did you get seven to nine hours of uninterrupted sleep?

- Are there physiological factors present, such as hormonal fluctuations?

- Are you adequately hydrated?

- Did something in your day create frustration or stress?

- Is there a conversation needing to happen with your spouse/partner/child/co-worker?

Cravings, like hunger, aren't signs of weakness or failure. They represent valuable and vital messages designed to help you find balance.

This journey ultimately returns to trusting your body's wisdom instead of ignoring what are natural, biological, and psychological processes of being human.

Embracing Food Freedom: The Healthy Eater Within

I'm frequently asked what constitutes a "normal eater." [1] I believe such a person doesn't exist; it's too broad a term and highly nuanced. Instead, we can become healthy eaters, those who cultivate a peaceful relationship with food rather than those who merely consume "perfectly healthy" foods.

Some of us thrive with three daily meals, while others prefer four to six smaller ones. Some comfortably skip meals when engaged in meaningful activities or confidently request specific preparations when dining out. Some maintain awareness of nutrition, while others simply enjoy what's available. Some occasionally overindulge during celebrations, while others rarely overeat because food holds different significance in their lives. Some prepare elaborate meals for loved ones, while others have local restaurants on speed dial.

All healthy eaters share these foundational practices:
- They honor their hunger and cravings with presence

---

1. (21) Koenig, Karen R. *The Rules of "Normal" Eating: A Commonsense Approach for Dieters, Overeaters, Undereaters, Emotional Eaters, and Everyone in Between!* Gurze Books, 2005.

- They choose foods that bring genuine satisfaction

- They eat with awareness, maintaining connection with their bodies

- They conclude their meals when feeling satisfied or comfortably full

I mentioned earlier that HOW we eat holds equal importance to WHAT we eat. Cultivating a nourishing relationship with food means we aren't defined by HOW much, HOW little, or HOW often we eat. Healthy eaters recognize and respond appropriately to their unique hunger signals.

By respecting their hunger, listening to what it's communicating, and including their bodies in this ongoing conversation, they choose truly satisfying nourishment. Healthy eaters don't select food based solely on calculating fat grams and calories. They don't wait until ravenous nor eat when not hungry. They make menu selections that appeal to them, not what someone across the table orders.

The empowering news is that we can relearn to attune ourselves to our body's wisdom and develop a healthier relationship with food as we begin to trust our hunger signals and, by extension, our bodies.

When we experience true satisfaction, we naturally stop when we've had enough. Feeling physically full and feeling genuinely satisfied represent separate but interconnected responses to hunger and the experience of eating. When we lose touch with our body's needs, discerning when we've had enough of anything, especially food, becomes challenging.

Often this disconnection stems from childhood messages about cleaning our plates because children were starving elsewhere or because our mothers labored over hot stoves. Perhaps your parents grew up during the Great Depression, teaching you to consume food quickly since scarcity loomed as a possibility. What happened was that as children, we weren't permitted to respond authentically to our body's signals for fullness and satisfaction. We matured into adults unable to recognize such signals, or we deliberately ignored them. We learned to base our sense of "enough" on external cues—portion sizes, whatever we could consume without consequences, what we believed we deserved, media influences, or even the approval of our dining companions.

Perhaps you felt pressure to maintain a certain weight to gain acceptance into your dream sorority; maybe childhood messages suggested no one would love you unless you were thin enough; perhaps your partner has indicated diminished attraction to larger bodies; maybe your weight offers protection from being fully seen and heard; maybe you've restricted yourself to a weight that makes you feel either invisible or powerful. In our quest for safety, love, and belonging, we often manipulate our nourishment patterns to achieve what we desire.

By not honoring our hunger authentically, we lose perspective on the greater truth—that what we're ultimately seeking is nourishment that reflects how we wish to experience life in its fullness.

You can begin cultivating a peaceful relationship with food by giving yourself unconditional permission to eat anything. This may sound counterintuitive, but when we remove moral judgments from our meal planning and snack choices, we liberate ourselves from the shame and guilt that emerge from relying solely on willpower. The next step involves trusting your hunger and fullness cues. The third step means eating primarily for physical rather than emotional reasons.

Making decisions about when and what to eat based on your body's authentic experiences creates profound empowerment. This empowerment emerges from asking yourself whether the food you're choosing will truly satisfy and sustain you. It's empowering to be accountable to the experience you desire from each meal. For example, if you're hungry for lunch and considering a smoothie, will it nourish you until your next meal? Would a salad alone provide satisfaction, or would adding protein create greater contentment? This mindful practice extends to foods typically on your "should not eat" list. If you have a sweet tooth, will fresh berries satisfy, or is a small portion of chocolate calling to you?

Because how we approach one aspect of life often mirrors how we approach everything, your relationship with food reflects how you work, connect with others, and care for yourself. Not recognizing when you've had enough may indicate uncertainty about effectively using the words "yes" and "no"—most evidently in your relationship with food. The restrictive eater says "no" too frequently; the emotional eater says "yes" too often. The goal is cultivating beautiful balance.

There can be genuine discomfort in learning to say both "no" and "yes" to ourselves and others with confidence. Developing this capacity introduces you to integrity with yourself and inspires and motivates you toward the loving, joyful, and vibrantly healthy life you deserve and desire.

Embrace Your Hunger Wisdom

When you feel drawn to eat without physical hunger, gently ask yourself, "What am I truly hungry for?" Acknowledge that you might be craving connection when alone or solitude when surrounded by others. Practice being fully present, experiencing what's unfolding within you, stepping out of your thoughts and into your body's wisdom. If your desire can be satisfied by something apart from food, it isn't physical hunger. Being totally present can be challenging for some people. If this is something you struggle with, seek support from a practitioner who will create a safe space for you to explore the context of this issue.

Remember that hunger represents an evolutionary survival mechanism. Even if you've disconnected from allowing yourself to experience physical hunger, trust that this wisdom remains within you. Before eating, create an intuitive inner scale from one to five. Level one represents the first whisper of hunger, while five signals intense hunger. Plan to nourish yourself when you reach levels two to three. Food tastes most exquisite when you're moderately hungry.

Learn to recognize when you've received enough nourishment by creating a fullness scale from one to five. Pause when you reach levels three to four , where you feel nourished and energized, satisfied but not uncomfortable. At this point, place your utensils down or, when appropriate, leave the table (without abandoning your companions). When dining out, request that your plate be removed or leftovers be packaged to take home. This will eliminate any visual cues for continued eating.

Your body's wisdom has been evolving for thousands of years. By reconnecting with these ancient signals, you reclaim the power to nourish yourself in ways that honor both your physical needs and your deepest hungers for a fully expressed life.

Chapter Summary

In this chapter, we explored the fundamental importance of reconnecting with our body's hunger signals as a pathway to food freedom. I distinguished between three types of hunger: physical hunger (our body's evolutionary wisdom), emotional hunger (our heart's yearning), and toxic hunger (our body's protest against nutritionally empty foods).

I shared my personal experience of restricting food during the day only to overeat in the evenings, illustrating how ignoring our body's signals creates the very behaviors we're trying to avoid. The chapter emphasizes that cravings aren't signs of weakness but rather important messengers about our physical, emotional, and spiritual needs. By learning to honor our hunger with presence, choosing foods that bring genuine satisfaction, eating with awareness, and stopping when comfortably full, we can cultivate a peaceful relationship with food that nourishes both our bodies and our souls.

Personal Reflection Exercises

Exercise 1: Hunger Awareness Mapping

For 3-5 days, create a personal hunger awareness map by tracking your hunger and fullness sensations throughout the day:

Create a simple tracking sheet with these columns:

- Time

- Hunger level (1-5 scale: 1 = first whisper of hunger, 5 = intense hunger)

- What I ate/drank

- Fullness level after eating (1-5 scale: 1 = still hungry, 5 = uncomfortably full)

- Physical sensations in my body (before and after eating)

- Emotions present

- Environment/circumstances

After completing your tracking period, reflect on these questions:

- When during the day do you typically first notice hunger?

- What patterns do you notice around your hunger and

fullness levels?

- How does your environment affect your eating patterns?

- What emotions most commonly accompany your eating experiences?

- When did you feel most satisfied after eating? What factors contributed to this satisfaction?

- When did you eat comfortably past fullness? What circumstances surrounded these instances?

Exercise 2: Distinguishing Your Three Hungers

Create a personal reference guide to help you recognize and respond appropriately to different types of hunger:

For each type of hunger, note:

Physical Hunger:

- How does it manifest in your body? (Specific sensations, locations, intensity)

- How gradually or suddenly does it develop?

- What foods typically satisfy it?

- How does your body feel when you respond appropriately?

Emotional Hunger:

- Which emotions most commonly trigger a desire to eat for you?

- What specific foods do you crave when emotionally hungry?

- What situations or relationships tend to trigger emotional eating?

- What non-food responses might better address these emotional needs?

Toxic Hunger:

- Which symptoms from the chapter do you recognize in your own experience?

- What foods or eating patterns seem to trigger these symptoms for you?

- How does toxic hunger feel different from true physical hunger?

- What whole-food alternatives might satisfy similar taste preferences?

Keep this reference guide accessible (perhaps in your phone or a small notebook) to consult when you're uncertain about what type of hunger you're experiencing.

Exercise 3: Craving Investigation Practice

Select one recurring food craving you experience and explore it with curiosity rather than judgment:

1. Document the Craving:

- What specific food do you crave?

- When does this craving typically occur? (Time of day, circumstances, etc.)

- What sensations accompany it? (Where in your body do you feel it?)

- What emotions are present when it arises?

2. Explore Possible Messages:

- Nutritional: What nutrients might your body be seeking? (Research nutrient content of craved foods)

- Emotional: What feelings might you be trying to soothe or enhance?

- Energetic: Is your body seeking specific energy (quick energy from sugar, sustained energy from fat, etc.)?

- Symbolic: What might this food represent in your life history or emotional landscape?

1. **Experiment with Responses:**

- Try satisfying the craving directly (eating the food with presence and enjoyment)

- Try satisfying potential nutritional needs with whole-food alternatives

- Try addressing emotional needs through non-food responses

- Compare how each response affects your satisfaction and well-being

Remember, the goal isn't to eliminate cravings but to understand their wisdom and respond in ways that truly nourish you.

Exercise 4: Permission Practice

This exercise helps release the restriction-rebellion cycle by exploring what unconditional permission to eat might feel like:

1. **List Your "Forbidden" Foods:**

- Write down foods you typically avoid, restrict, or feel guilty about eating

- For each food, note when you first categorized it as bad or off-limits

- Reflect on messages you received about this food

(from family, media, diet culture, etc.)

2. Choose One "Forbidden" Food for Exploration:

- Purchase a small amount of this food when you're not extremely hungry

- Create a calm, distraction-free environment

- Before eating, acknowledge any guilt, fear, or anxiety that arises

- Give yourself full permission to eat and enjoy this food

3. Practice Mindful Enjoyment:

- Observe the food with all your senses before taking the first bite

- Eat slowly, savoring each bite fully

- Pause halfway through to check in with your satisfaction and fullness

- Continue until you feel satisfied (not deprived, not uncomfortably full)

4. Reflection After the Experience:

- How did the actual experience compare to your anticipation of it?

- Did the food taste as good as you expected throughout the experience?

- At what point did satisfaction begin to diminish?

- What emotions arose before, during, and after eating?

This isn't a one-time exercise but a practice to repeat with different foods as you build trust with your body and decrease the emotional charge around formerly "forbidden" foods.

Journal Prompts

1. **Hunger History:** Reflect on your earliest memories of hunger. How was hunger viewed in your family? Were you encouraged to honor your hunger or ignore it? How were messages about ignoring fullness communicated? How have these early experiences shaped your current relationship with hunger?

2. **Satisfaction Exploration:** Describe a recent meal that felt truly satisfying. What elements contributed to this satisfaction? Consider the food itself, your hunger level, the environment, your emotional state, and the company (if any). How might you incorporate more of these satisfaction elements into your daily eating?

3. **Hunger-Fullness Disconnection:** I shared how I would restrict myself throughout the day only to overeat in the

evening. Does this pattern sound familiar? If so, explore how ignoring your hunger throughout the day affects your evening eating. What beliefs or fears keep you from honoring earlier hunger signals?

4. **Beyond Food Nourishment:** Consider the question: "Are you hearing, 'I need chocolate' when what you're truly seeking might be spirituality, sensuality, movement, joy, or creative expression?" What non-food forms of nourishment might your heart and spirit be craving right now? How might you begin to fulfill these deeper hungers?

5. **Yes and No Boundaries:** Reflect on the observation that "The restrictive eater says 'no' too frequently; the emotional eater says 'yes' too often." Where in your relationship with food do you need to practice saying "yes" more confidently? Where might you need to practice a loving "no"? How might finding this balance affect other areas of your life?

Practice: The Hunger-Fullness Scale Experiment

This week, practice using the intuitive hunger-fullness scale mentioned in the chapter to guide your eating decisions:

Preparation:

1. Create a small card or note in your phone with these

scales:

- **Hunger Scale:** 1 (first whisper of hunger) to 5 (intense hunger)

- **Fullness Scale:** 1 (still hungry) to 5 (uncomfortably full)

2. Post visual reminders in places where you typically make food decisions (kitchen, dining area, inside your planner, etc.)

Daily Practice:
1. **Before Eating:**

- Take 3 deep breaths to center yourself

- Scan your body and rate your current hunger level (1-5)

- Ask yourself: "What would truly satisfy me right now?"

- Make your food choice based on this awareness

2. **During Eating:**

- Pause after every few bites

- Notice flavors, textures, and your enjoyment level

○ Check in with your hunger/fullness sensations

3. **After Eating:**

○ Rate your fullness level (1-5)

○ Note your energy and satisfaction level

○ Reflect on what you learned from this eating experience

Remember:

- Aim to begin eating when you reach levels 2-3 on the hunger scale

- Aim to stop eating when you reach levels 3-4 on the fullness scale

- There are no "wrong" answers—this is about developing awareness, not judgment

- If you eat when not hungry or past comfortable fullness, simply note it with curiosity

Weekly Reflection: At the end of the week, review your experiences:

- When were you most successful at eating in response to moderate hunger?

- What factors made it challenging to honor your hunger

and fullness cues?

- How did eating at different hunger and fullness levels affect your energy, mood, and satisfaction?

- What one insight will you carry forward into the next week?

Craving Response Toolkit

Create a personal toolkit for responding mindfully to your cravings:

For Each Common Craving Type, Identify:

Sweet Cravings:

- Possible nutritional needs (protein, complex carbs, chromium, etc.)

- Whole-food options that satisfy sweet taste (fruit, sweet vegetables, etc.)

- Non-food sweetness for your life (joy, pleasure, rest, etc.)

- Mindful indulgence options when a treat is truly desired

Salty Cravings:

- Possible nutritional needs (minerals, electrolytes, etc.)

- Nourishing salty food options (nuts, seeds, broths, etc.)

- What saltiness might represent emotionally (grounded-ness, vitality, etc.)

- How to address any mineral deficiencies through whole foods

Comfort Food Cravings:
- The emotions typically driving these cravings

- The memories or associations with these foods

- Non-food comforts that might address the emotional need

- Ways to honor the emotional significance while nourish-ing your body

Create a Physical Resource: Compile your insights into a reference guide (a special section in your journal, a note in your phone, or a small physical card) that you can consult when cravings arise. Include:
- Quick assessment questions to identify hunger type

- Options for responding to each craving type

- Reminders of what different cravings might be telling you

- Compassionate phrases to use with yourself during chal-lenging moments

Keep this toolkit accessible and refine it as you discover what works best for you.

"What Am I Hungry For?" Meditation

This guided reflection helps you develop deeper awareness of your various hungers:

Find a comfortable seated position and close your eyes. Take 3 deep breaths, feeling your body relax with each exhale.

1. **Physical Body Scan:**

   ○ Bring awareness to your physical body, starting at your feet and moving upward

   ○ Notice any sensations in your stomach, chest, and throat

   ○ Is there physical emptiness, rumbling, or energy depletion?

   ○ Simply observe these sensations without judgment

2. **Emotional Landscape:**

   ○ Shift your awareness to your emotional state

   ○ What emotions are present for you right now?

   ○ Is there loneliness, boredom, anxiety, joy, or something else?

- Notice where in your body you feel these emotions

3. **Heart and Spirit:**

- Move your attention to deeper yearnings

- What might your heart be hungry for? Connection? Expression? Purpose?

- What might your spirit be craving? Meaning? Beauty? Transcendence?

- Allow these deeper hungers to reveal themselves without forcing

4. **Integrated Awareness:**

- As you integrate all these levels of awareness, ask yourself:

- "What am I truly hungry for at this moment?"

- Wait patiently for the answer to emerge

- Notice if the answer surprises you

5. **Compassionate Response:**

- Consider what would most nourish you right now

- This might be food, rest, connection, expression, or something else

- Set an intention to respond to your true hunger with kindness

6. Close by placing 1 hand on your heart and 1 hand on your belly, acknowledging the wisdom of both.

Practice this meditation when you feel drawn to food but aren't sure if you're physically hungry. With practice, you'll develop greater clarity about your various hungers and how to nourish them appropriately.

Looking Forward

As you continue your journey through *Midlife Metamorphosis*, notice how honoring your hunger creates a foundation for the food freedom you're cultivating. When you trust your body's signals, you establish a relationship with food based on respect and attunement rather than fear and control. This reconnection with your body's wisdom builds upon the emotional awareness work from previous chapters and prepares you for deeper exploration of nourishment beyond food.

Remember that reclaiming your hunger wisdom is a practice, not a perfect science. Some days will flow more easily than others. What matters most is your willingness to keep listening and to approach your body's messages with curiosity and compassion rather than judgment.

"By reconnecting with these ancient signals, you reclaim the power to nourish yourself in ways that honor both your physical needs and your deepest hungers for a fully expressed life." - Mindy

Embrace Movement That Nurtures

Honoring Your Body's Wisdom

Finding Your Way to Movement That Celebrates You

D o you move your body from a place of deep reverence and celebration or from fear and judgment?

This question invites us to explore the profound difference between exercise as punishment and movement as liberation.

My journey with movement reflects the transformation many of us experience in midlife. For years, I chased the validation of personal trainers whose approval I sought through physical transformation. Each class, each session, became another opportunity to prove my worth through my body's appearance rather than its inherent wisdom and strength.

A turning point came unexpectedly when an accident left me with a serious shoulder injury. The orthopedist noted that my regular exercise had created strength that prevented more severe damage. This moment offered my first glimpse of my training's true gift—not as a tool for changing my appearance, but as a practice that builds strength, resilience, and nurtures well-being.

Yet old patterns persist. Even as I recovered, I found myself gravitating toward trainers who pushed me to exhaustion, mistaking intensity for worth. One kept garbage pails nearby for clients who pushed themselves to vomit, a stark reminder of how disconnected we can become from our bodies' wisdom when we prioritize transformation over attunement.

Another lesson learned...

In the early nineties, I discovered the StairMaster. I had been exercising for a few years when Olivia Newton-John had the hit single "Let's Get Physical." I had no clue as to the benefits of exercise. Embodiment and endorphins were concepts that were foreign to me. What I did relate to was that the more I exercised, the more calories I would burn, and the skinnier I could become. If I were really diligent, I could actually experience a calorie deficit in my day.

On one trip, we were visiting my parents in Florida. They lived in a gated country club community that boasted a state-of-the-art gym. Treadmills were built into the floor, and Stairmasters^{TM} and stair-climbing machines were recently installed. I had read somewhere that the Stairmasters™ could burn the most calories and have a great effect on your thighs. Sign me up.

Every day, for one hour, I would escape to the gym and climb my way to thigh nirvana. When we returned home, I talked my husband into buying a home model. About a month into my routine, I discovered that all my pants were getting tighter. Devastated, I decided to eat less and exercise more. Little did I know that the very machine I was counting on to make my body go away was contributing to muscle growth, and my thighs were getting bigger. It was as though a sick joke was being played on me. Lesson learned. Our bodies are unique and respond as such. What works for some may not be appropriate for all.

The journey toward embodiment requires us to release the weight of perfectionism. When I finally allowed myself to step away from punishing routines, I discovered movement that felt like coming home. Walking outdoors with friends and practicing Pilates™ and yoga became pathways to presence, not escape. I found instructors who respected the wisdom of a maturing body and approached movement with reverence for what is, rather than fixation on what should be.

This shift represents the heart of what I hope to share with you: movement as a celebration of life rather than a correction of perceived flaws. True freedom from an unhealthy relationship with food cannot happen without our ability and willingness to connect with our bodies. When we listen to what our bodies tell us, we naturally gravitate toward movement that helps us thrive.

Honoring Our Changing Bodies in Midlife

As we journey through midlife, our bodies tell the stories of our lives—the joys, the sorrows, the transformations. Yet society often teaches us to wage war against these natural changes, selling us products and procedures promising to erase the visible markers of our experience.

The silver strands weaving through our hair, the laugh lines framing our eyes, the laxity of our skin—these are not flaws to be corrected but testaments to a life fully lived. Each mark, each change, carries wisdom gained through experience.

Many women in their fifties, sixties, and beyond describe feeling invisible in a culture that celebrates youth above all else. Yet this invisibility can become a radical opportunity for freedom, the freedom from the exhausting pursuit of external validation, the freedom to inhabit our bodies with newfound authenticity.

The softening of our belly that once carried children or weathered stress, the changing landscape of our skin that has protected us through decades of living, the bones that may grow more delicate yet have supported us through countless journeys—these deserve our respect and gratitude, not our criticism.

When I speak with women about their changing bodies, I often hear painful reflections:

"I avoid looking in the mirror when I step out of the shower."

"I feel betrayed by my body. It doesn't look or move the way it once did."

"I spend so much energy trying to hide the parts of me that show my age."

This distress isn't surprising in a world that bombards us with anti-aging messages. Messages that aging is something to be fought at all costs. But what if we could embrace another perspective? What if these changes are not something to resist, but rather transformations, not diminishment, but evolution?

Our bodies in midlife reflect profound courage. The skin that sags has elasticity that allowed us to grow children or weather weight fluctuations. The wrinkles around our eyes have witnessed both tears of sorrow and laughter reflecting pure joy. Even the aches in our joints speak to years of movement by dancing and carrying those we love.

This perspective doesn't deny the real challenges of aging. Bone density may decrease, making mindful strength training more important. Hormonal shifts may change how our bodies distribute weight or respond to certain foods. Sleep patterns may shift, and bouncing back from injury or exertion may take longer.

But these changes invite us into a more aligned relationship with our bodies rather than a more combative one. They ask us to listen more carefully, to honor our limitations while still exploring our capabilities, and to practice patience and compassion where we might once have demanded perfection.

The Power of Your Inner Voice

The relationship we have with our bodies begins in our minds. The thoughts we cultivate and the words we speak to ourselves create the foundation for how we experience embodiment.

Consider for a moment how you speak to someone you deeply love. You likely choose words that uplift, encourage, and recognize their inherent worth. Now, reflect on how you speak to your body. Do you offer the same compassion and respect? Or do you criticize, compare, and find fault?

This recognition can be uncomfortable, but it opens the door to transformation. Self-affirmation—the practice of consciously choosing supportive, empowering thoughts—creates a foundation for healing. As psychologist Claude Steele's research shows, we have a fundamental need to maintain self-integrity and perceive ourselves as worthy and capable. When we align our thoughts with this truth, we begin to experience our bodies differently. [1]

Start with simple affirmations that challenge your habitual negative thoughts:

I am beginning to accept myself more each day.

I am overcoming negative patterns and building a positive relationship with my body.

---

1. Steele, C. M. (1988). The psychology of self-affirmation: Sustaining the integrity of the self. Advances in Experimental Social Psychology, 21, 261-302. https://doi.org/10.1016/S0 065-2601(08)60229-4

I am grateful for my body and all it does for me.

My body deserves respect and care.

I appreciate my [specific quality] and how it serves me.

At first, these words may feel foreign or even false. Remember that you are challenging years of conditioned thinking. Start with one statement that feels authentic, and allow it to take root in your consciousness. With time and practice, these new thoughts will become your natural way of being.

Movement as Embodiment

Movement is not merely something we do; it's a way of inhabiting our bodies with presence and wisdom. Our bodies are designed for movement—they crave it, thrive on it, and deteriorate without it.

The physiological benefits of regular movement extend far beyond weight management:

- **Rejuvenation**: Regular cardiovascular activity improves oxygen intake, effectively reducing biological age.

- **Immune Support**: Even moderate exercise temporarily enhances immune function, reducing susceptibility to illness.

- **Heart Health**: Movement improves cholesterol levels, lowers blood pressure, and reduces arterial inflammation.

- **Respiratory Wellness**: Upper body and breathing exercises can improve symptoms of asthma and enhance lung capacity.

- **Metabolic Balance**: Regular walking helps regulate blood sugar and improves insulin sensitivity.

- **Cancer Prevention**: Exercise may reduce the risk of several cancers through hormone regulation and improved digestion.

- **Stress Relief**: Movement lowers stress hormones and releases endorphins that enhance emotional well-being.

- **Menopausal Support**: Walking and gentle yoga can reduce hot flashes and night sweats.

- **Bone Strength**: Weight-bearing exercises help maintain bone density, particularly crucial during and after menopause.

- **Joint Health**: Gentle movement lubricates joints and builds supporting muscles, easing discomfort and improving mobility.

These benefits support long-term health and vitality. Yet many of us approach exercise as another form of escape, punishment, or compensation for eating behaviors we've labeled as indulgent. This mindset is no different from the restrictive mentality that drives chronic dieting.

The media landscape perpetuates this disconnection, with celebrity trainers and influencers promoting extreme routines that leave us feeling inadequate if we don't keep up and spend hours in the gym. These messages are especially harmful if you already struggle with body image. When exercise becomes something you *should* do rather than something you enjoy doing, it creates a stress response that undermines the very benefits you seek.

Conversely, you may avoid movement altogether, believing you must first resolve your weight or self-esteem issues before you can engage with your body. Either approach creates a no-win situation where limiting beliefs prevent you from experiencing the joy of embodiment.

When we shift from punishing exercise to pleasurable movement, we honor our bodies' inherent wisdom. This shift naturally leads to more nourishing food choices and a sense of vitality that is both energizing and grounding.

Finding Your Unique Movement Practice

Clients often ask about the "best" time and type of exercise. The truth is that the best approach is the one that resonates with your body and lifestyle. Some women feel most energized in the morning, while others find their rhythm in the evening. Different forms of movement offer different benefits, and your preferences may change with the seasons of your life.

Consider what draws you to movement:

- Do you thrive on the connection in team sports?

- Does a skilled instructor inspire you in a group setting?

- Do you prefer the solitude of home practice?

- Does being outdoors rejuvenate your spirit?

The possibilities are endless when pleasure and well-being become your guiding principles.

Movement connects you to the sensations of being alive when you approach it with curiosity rather than judgment. This connection builds trust in your body's wisdom and frees you from external measures of worth, like the scale—a device whose sole purpose is to keep you tied to numbers rather than sensations.

When you focus on how food "will affect you" or how exercise "will change you," you miss the chance to appreciate your body's beauty and brilliance, such as the legs that ground you, the arms that let you hug loved ones, the belly that guides you with intuition or perhaps carries life.

Embracing Your Body's History

Our bodies in midlife carry the sacred text of our experience—stretch marks that testify to growth, scars that commemorate healing, and lines that map our emotional landscapes. In a culture that has taught women to apologize for taking up space, minimize our presence, and erase our histories from our skin, the simple act of honoring these markers becomes revolutionary.

Consider the power of touching your body with reverence rather than criticism. What might change if you placed your hands on your softening midsection with gratitude for how it has protected your vital organs throughout your life? If you viewed the lines on your face as tributaries of expression instead of eliminating them as flaws, what might change?

One of my clients, Maria, shared a profound transformation in her relationship with her body after decades of self-criticism. At fifty-eight, she had spent years avoiding swimming, an activity she once loved, because she felt ashamed of her changing body. Through our work together, she began a simple practice of thanking her body each night for specific ways it had served her that day.

"Thank you, legs, for carrying me through my workday."

"Thank you, hands, for creating beautiful meals and holding my grandchild."

"Thank you, heart, for continuing to beat faithfully through joy and sorrow."

This practice gradually shifted her perspective. Six months later, she sent me a photo of herself in a swimsuit, beaming alongside her grandchildren at the beach. "I realized I was teaching them to fear and dishonor a changing body," she wrote. "Now I'm teaching them to experience joy in every chapter of life."

This doesn't mean the journey is linear or that cultural messaging suddenly loses its power. Rather, it means we commit to returning, again and again, to this practice of honoring our bodies' wisdom and history, recognizing that each time we do, we strengthen our capacity for self-compassion and embodied presence.

Embracing Embodiment

Improving body image in midlife requires a compassionate, multifaceted approach, especially when integrating movement. Consider these strategies:

- Focus on joy rather than calorie-burning or aesthetic goals

- Practice mindfulness through activities that enhance body awareness

- Set feeling-based goals related to energy, stress reduction, or relaxation

- Embrace body neutrality by appreciating function over appearance

- Create safe spaces for movement without comparison or judgment

- Incorporate restorative practices that promote ease and relaxation

- Honor your autonomy by choosing movements that feel right for you

- Cultivate body awareness through somatic practices

without criticism

- Use affirming language that challenges negative self-perception

- Integrate supportive practices like coaching or community support

The ultimate goal is to develop a relationship with movement that promotes healing and strengthens body image without perpetuating patterns of disordered eating or negative self-perception.

Your Invitation to Embodiment

Today, I invite you to try a new, enjoyable activity that helps you feel connected to your body. Notice how it feels to move from a place of curiosity rather than criticism.

As an advanced practice, consider gentle mirror work. Stand before a mirror, clothed or not, and allow yourself to discover your beauty, part by part. As you do, repeat affirming statements:

I am beginning to accept myself more each day.

I am building a positive relationship with my body.

I am grateful for what my body can do.

My body deserves respect and appreciation.

I appreciate my [specific quality].

Write these statements on cards and place them where they'll remind you of your commitment to self-compassion. If you find it challenging to identify positive qualities, invite a trusted friend or family member to share what they appreciate about you.

Remember that this body—this miraculous vessel that has carried you through every triumph and heartbreak, every celebration and challenge—deserves your kindness. It has never stopped working for you, even when you were at war with it. Perhaps now, in this season of life, is the perfect time to declare peace and establish a new relationship based on respect, appreciation, and joy.

Chapter Summary

In this chapter, we explore the paradigm shift from viewing exercise as punishment to embracing movement as a celebration of life. I share my personal journey from using exercise as a tool for changing my appearance to discovering movement as a practice that builds resilience and nurtures well-being. The chapter addresses the unique challenges and opportunities of our changing midlife bodies, emphasizing that the visible markers of our experience are not flaws to be corrected but testaments to lives fully lived.

You learned the immense physical and emotional benefits of regular movement while challenging the harmful messaging that promotes extreme routines or punishment-based exercise. I encourage you to develop a relationship with movement based on pleasure, attunement, and respect for our bodies' inherent wisdom. The chapter concludes with an invitation to approach our bodies with reverence rather than criticism, recognizing that our midlife bodies carry the sacred text of our existence and deserve our gratitude and compassion.

Personal Reflection Exercises

Exercise 1: Your Movement History Timeline

Create a visual timeline of your relationship with movement throughout your life:

1. Draw a horizontal line across a page, marking different life stages (childhood, teens, 20s, 30s, 40s, 50s, etc.).

2. For each life stage, note:

   ○ Types of movement you engaged in

   ○ Your feelings about your body during this time

   ○ What motivated your movement choices

   ○ Whether movement felt like celebration or punishment

   ○ Any significant events that affected your relationship with movement

3. Looking at your timeline as a whole, reflect:

   ○ When was movement most joyful for you?

   ○ When did it feel most disconnected from pleasure?

- What patterns do you notice in your relationship with movement?

- What insights does this history offer about your current approach to movement?

Exercise 2: Movement Motivation Inventory

This exercise helps clarify your current motivations for movement and invites a shift toward more nurturing intentions.

Create three columns on a page:

Column 1: My Current Movement Motivations

List all the reasons you currently move your body or think you "should" move your body. Be completely honest and include appearance-based motivations, health concerns, fears, external pressures, etc.

Column 2: The Emotional Experience These Create

For each motivation, note how it makes you feel emotionally. Does it generate pressure, anxiety, shame, empowerment, peace, etc.?

Column 3: More Nurturing Motivations

For each of your current motivations, craft a more nurturing alternative that honors your body's wisdom. For example:

- "To burn calories" might become "To experience energy flowing through my body"

- "To fix my problem areas" might become "To appreciate

what my body can do"

- "Because I should" might become "To connect with my body's natural desire for movement"

Select 2-3 nurturing motivations that resonate most deeply with you. Write these on small cards and place them where you'll see them before engaging in movement.

Exercise 3: Body Appreciation Practice

This exercise helps develop awareness of your body's capabilities rather than focusing on its appearance:

1. Create a body gratitude list with these categories:

    ○ Things my body allows me to experience (sensations, pleasures, connections)

    ○ Ways my body has carried me through challenges

    ○ Activities my body enables me to enjoy

    ○ How my body communicates its needs to me

    ○ Reasons I'm grateful for specific parts of my body (based on function, not appearance)

2. Choose one area of your body that you typically criticize. Write a letter of appreciation to this part, acknowledging how it has served you throughout your life. For example,

a letter to your belly might acknowledge how it:

- Houses and protects vital organs

- Perhaps carried children

- Digests the food that nourishes you

- Holds wisdom in your gut feelings

- Bears the marks of your life experiences

3. Create a simple ritual to express gratitude to your body daily. This might be placing your hands on your heart before sleep, thanking specific body parts during your shower, or acknowledging your body's service before movement.

Exercise 4: Movement Pleasure Exploration

This exercise helps you discover (or rediscover) forms of movement that bring genuine pleasure:

1. Brainstorm a diverse list of movement options, being as creative and open-minded as possible. Include activities from your past that brought joy, movements you've been curious about, and options that feel accessible for your current body.

2. Rate each option on a pleasure potential scale of 1-10,

based on your intuition about how enjoyable it might be.

3. Select three options with high pleasure potential that you could realistically try in the next month.

4. For each selected option, identify:

   ○ What you would need to make this possible (equipment, clothing, instruction, childcare, etc.)

   ○ Any barriers that might prevent you from trying it

   ○ One small step you could take this week toward making it happen

5. Commit to trying at least one new form of movement this month with the explicit intention of discovering pleasure rather than achieving any specific outcome.

After trying each new movement, journal about:

- Physical sensations you noticed

- Emotional responses that arose

- Aspects you enjoyed or found challenging

- Whether you'd like to incorporate this movement into your life regularly

Journal Prompts

1. **Movement as Celebration:** Do you move your body from a place of deep reverence and celebration or from fear and judgment? Reflect honestly on this question. What might shift in your experience if you approached movement as a celebration of what your body can do rather than an attempt to change it?

2. **Midlife Body Changes:** The chapter describes how our bodies in midlife "tell the stories of our lives—the joys, the sorrows, the transformations." What stories does your body tell? How might viewing bodily changes as transformations rather than diminishment affect how you experience aging?

3. **Inner Voice Awareness:** Consider how you speak to your body during or after movement. What specific phrases or thoughts arise? If you were to speak to your body as you would to someone you deeply love, what would you say instead?

4. **Movement Benefits Beyond Appearance:** The chapter lists numerous benefits of movement beyond weight management. Which of these benefits resonates most strongly with you personally? How might focusing on these benefits, rather than appearance, change your rela-

tionship with movement?

5. **Embodied Presence:** Reflect on a time when you felt fully present and at home in your body. What were you doing? What conditions helped create this sense of embodiment? How might you cultivate more of these experiences in your daily life?

Practice: Movement for Pleasure Experiment

This week, commit to approaching movement with the primary goal of pleasure and body connection.

Preparation:

1. Release any appearance-related goals for this experiment

2. Set an intention to discover what types of movement bring you genuine joy

3. Give yourself full permission to modify or stop any activity that doesn't feel good in your body

Daily Practice (15-30 minutes):

1. **Check-In:** Before moving, take three deep breaths and ask your body what kind of movement it desires today. Options might include:

   ○ Gentle stretching or yoga

   ○ Walking outdoors

- Dancing to favorite music

- Swimming or water movement

- Gardening or household tasks that involve pleasant movement

- Playful movement (throwing a ball, hula hooping, jumping rope)

- Flowing movement like tai chi or qigong

- Strength-building movements that feel empowering

2. **Mindful Engagement:**

- Move slowly enough to notice physical sensations

- Focus on how the movement feels rather than how you look

- Express gratitude to your body for its capabilities

- Adjust any movement that causes pain or discomfort

- Notice moments of pleasure or satisfaction

3. **Reflection:**

- After moving, take a moment to acknowledge how your body feels

- ○ Note any shifts in your energy, mood, or physical sensations

- ○ Thank your body for this experience

Weekly Integration: At the end of the week, reflect on your experiences:

- Which forms of movement brought the most pleasure?

- What conditions (time of day, environment, music, etc.) enhanced your enjoyment?

- How did approaching movement for pleasure affect your overall relationship with your body?

- What insights from this experiment would you like to carry forward?

Remember that this is an experiment in awareness, not a new regimen to perfect. The goal is simply to reconnect with your body's inherent desire for joyful movement.

Mirror Compassion Practice

As mentioned in the chapter, mirror work can be a powerful practice for developing self-compassion. This exercise offers a gentle approach to this practice:

Begin with Preparation:

- Choose a time when you won't be interrupted

- Create a calming environment (perhaps with soft lighting, music, or a candle)

- Have your affirmation cards nearby

- Remind yourself that this practice may bring up emotions, all of which are welcome

The Practice

1. **Grounding:** Stand or sit comfortably before a mirror. Take three deep breaths.

2. **Gentle Gaze:** Meet your own eyes with softness. If this feels too intense, you can begin by looking at your hands in the mirror.

3. **Compassionate Presence:** Imagine looking at a dear friend who has shared their body insecurities with you. What would you say to them? How would you look at them?

4. **Part-by-Part Appreciation:** Moving slowly from head to toe, acknowledge each part of your body with gratitude for its function:

   ○ "Thank you, eyes, for allowing me to see beauty in the world."

   ○ "Thank you, shoulders, for carrying my burdens and for the ability to embrace those I love."

- "Thank you, heart, for continuing to beat faithfully through joy and sorrow."

- Continue with each part of your body, focusing on function rather than appearance

5. **Whole-Self Acknowledgment:** Looking at your whole self, repeat one of your chosen affirmations:

   - "I am beginning to accept myself more each day."

   - "I am building a positive relationship with my body."

   - "I am grateful for what my body can do."

   - "My body deserves respect and appreciation."

6. **Closure:** Place your hand on your heart, take a deep breath, and silently acknowledge the courage it takes to practice this kind of compassion.

Begin with just 2-3 minutes and gradually extend the practice as it becomes more comfortable. If looking in the mirror feels too challenging initially, you can start by practicing with a photograph of yourself, preferably one where you appear happy and relaxed.

Movement Wisdom Circle (Group Practice)

This practice is designed for group settings, creating a safe space to share experiences and wisdom about nurturing movement.

Preparation:

- Arrange chairs in a circle

- Have a talking piece (a stone, feather, or other meaningful object)

- Establish group agreements: confidentiality, non-judgment, speaking from personal experience, and listening with compassion

Opening:

- The facilitator briefly introduces the concept of movement as celebration rather than punishment

- Participants take three collective breaths to center themselves in the present moment

Sharing Rounds:

1. **Memory Round:** Share a memory of a time when movement brought you joy. (Each person shares briefly while holding the talking piece)

2. **Wisdom Round:** What has your body taught you through movement that you couldn't have learned any other way?

3. **Challenge Round:** What harmful messages about exercise or movement do you have, and how are you releasing them?

4. **Vision Round:** What would a truly nurturing relationship with movement look like in your life going forward?

Integration:

- After all rounds, participants reflect together on common themes and insights

- Each person shares one small step they'll take in the coming week to move with more compassion and joy

Closing:

- The group stands in a circle and each person offers one word that represents what they're taking from the experience

- A final collective breath completes the practice

This circle creates space for collective wisdom to emerge while honoring each person's unique experience with movement and embodiment.

Looking Forward

As you continue your journey through *Midlife Metamorphosis*, notice how embracing nurturing movement complements the mindfulness practices from the previous chapter and supports your developing relationship with hunger and satisfaction. Movement that honors your body's wisdom naturally enhances your ability to recognize and respond to your body's signals around food, creating a virtuous cycle of embodied awareness.

Remember that transforming your relationship with movement, like transforming your relationship with food, is a practice of returning again and again to presence and compassion. Each time you choose a movement that celebrates rather than punishes your body, you strengthen your capacity for radical acceptance and deepen your connection to your body's inherent wisdom.

"Remember that this body—this miraculous vessel that has carried you through every triumph and heartbreak, every celebration and challenge—deserves your kindness. It has never stopped working for you, even when you were at war with it." - Mindy

Nourishment as Liberation

Your Journey to Food Freedom

"Let food be thy medicine, and medicine be thy food."

— Hippocrates

Dear friend, take a breath. In this moment, let's create a pause where you can gently release the weight of food fears you've carried for far too long. Perhaps use this time to imagine the lightness of being you will experience when those burdens are no longer weighing on you.

Like many women in this remarkable middle season of life, you've likely traveled down countless paths in search of the "perfect" way to eat. Perhaps you've counted calories until the numbers blurred, restricted carbs until your energy waned, or methodically measured protein at every meal. You may have embraced veganism, vegetarianism, gone gluten-free, dairy-free, or attempted to sustain yourself on smaller, more frequent meals throughout the day.

What these approaches share isn't health—it's disciplined constraint. They've boxed you into rigid rules, leaving you feeling like a failure when you inevitably step outside their arbitrary boundaries.

The truth? These rules emerged from belief systems, limited and limiting belief systems, that were never designed for your unique magnificence.

Beyond the Battle: Ending Your War with Food

This chapter is your invitation to freedom, to end the exhausting war with food that has consumed precious energy better spent on living your most vibrant life. Together, we'll continue to explore the science, psychology, and soulful wisdom that allows you to adopt a relaxed, intuitive relationship with nourishment, one where you can enjoy foods you love while you discover and explore connecting to their energy with a sense of calm.

Many of us fear food for complex reasons. Some fears originate in our personal histories. Others stem from what Marc David, founder of the Institute for the Psychology of Eating, calls "toxic nutritional beliefs"—ideas about eating that harm rather than heal. And some emerge from the dizzying array of conflicting advice from so-called experts telling us what to eat and what to avoid.

This brings me to sharing how I define disordered eating, a misguided behavior that is driven by misinformation.

The freedom I invite you to embrace comes from making choices fueled by a desire to feel your best, not from external rules. Often, you'll discover that what you believed was right for your body wasn't right at all. What's healthy for one woman can be inflammatory for another. True nourishment is deeply personal.

You might wonder, *How is this freedom if I'm not eating whatever I want?* I ask you to consider this: Where is the joy if what you're choosing leaves you feeling unwell? Can you reframe your beliefs about what truly satisfies? Can you see that self-indulgence masquerading as freedom often deprives you of becoming the woman you long to be?

The Midlife Table: Nourishment Through Transition

During midlife, our relationship with food often undergoes profound transformation. The body that could once seemingly process anything without complaint now speaks to us with more urgency and clarity. Such behavior isn't a betrayal, it's an invitation to deeper listening.

Sarah, a fifty-year-old client, described it beautifully. "For decades, I ate whatever was convenient, whatever fit into my busy schedule raising children and building my career. Now, my body has become like a wise elder; it speaks with authority about what truly nourishes me. When I listen, I feel vibrant. When I ignore its wisdom, I pay the price."

This midlife dialogue with our bodies isn't about restriction—it's about revelation. As hormones shift, our nutritional needs evolve. The metabolism that once burned with the fire of youth now asks for different fuel. Our digestive system may become more sensitive, our blood sugar stability more precarious, and our need for particular nutrients more pronounced.

These changes aren't failures or weaknesses but guideposts. They direct us toward nourishment that supports this magnificent transition, this powerful threshold we're crossing. When we approach these changes with curiosity rather than resistance, we discover a new kind of freedom, the freedom that comes from alignment with our body's deepest wisdom.

Honoring Your Unique Symphony: Bio-Individuality

My deepest hope is that you emerge from these pages with a renewed understanding of both the nutritional and spiritual dimensions of eating. I want you to develop curiosity about different foods and nutritional approaches, discovering what genuinely serves your body at this magnificent midlife moment.

Like many women I've worked with, you likely understand the latest nutritional science such as what's "in" and what's "out." Despite extensive dieting experience, you may still feel confused about what to eat, especially as your body changes through midlife.

Following trends or emulating someone with an entirely different body type will only lead to disappointment. Your unique physiology processes foods differently than anyone else's. If you've been restricting, bingeing, or purging, you're likely experiencing digestive distress and symptoms calling for attention.

> **Remember this fundamental truth that's based on a functional medicine philosophy: "We are not what we eat, but what our bodies do with what we eat." This belief is the cornerstone of functional nutrition. While certain dietary approaches work beautifully for me—supporting my energy, satisfaction, and overall wellness—they may not serve you.**

The answer is bio-individuality. There is no single "right" diet for every woman. Diets are not universally applicable. Today, and every day going forward, is your opportunity to honor your unique physiology and become the master of your physical, emotional, and mental well-being.

The Essential Elements: Understanding Macronutrients

Protein: Your Body's Building Blocks

Protein supplies the fundamental building blocks for every cell in your magnificent body. It's essential for maintaining muscle mass, which naturally begins to decrease in midlife, making adequate protein particularly crucial during this life stage.

High-quality proteins include organic meats and poultry, wild and conscientiously raised fish, whole soy foods, organic dairy, pasture-raised eggs, nuts, and seeds. When protein is insufficient—common among women who chronically diet—you might experience irritability, fatigue, poor memory, cravings, hair loss, brittle nails, digestive issues, feeling cold, poor muscle tone, and decreased libido.

Your protein needs may shift with the seasons and your life circumstances. During recovery from illness, periods of intense activity, or times of growth and change (including the transitions of midlife), your needs may increase.

A client of mine, Elena, struggled with afternoon energy crashes and persistent sugar cravings. When we gently increased her protein intake—adding a palm-sized portion to each meal—her energy stabilized and cravings diminished.

"I never realized how much my body was asking for protein," she told me. "I'd been ignoring its signals for years."

Carbohydrates: Embracing What You've Been Taught to Fear

Carbohydrates are necessary for balance and vitality; they provide energy that fuels your body and brain continuously. Your internal organs, nervous system, and muscles depend on carbohydrates to function. They help metabolize protein and fat and contain the fiber, vitamins, minerals, and enzymes needed for optimal well-being.

Carbohydrates encompass a wide spectrum of foods, from the sweetest honey to the most vibrant leafy greens. All fruits, vegetables, legumes, and grains are primarily carbohydrates, though they contain varying amounts of protein and fat.

While natural carbohydrates are essential, overly processed and refined versions offer no nutritional benefits. In fact, they deplete precious nutrients like magnesium, zinc, and B vitamins during digestion, essentially becoming "anti-nutrients." Examples of such would commercially baked and packaged products and mass-produced and marketed snack foods such as the vast array of chips available.

Carbohydrate needs differ significantly among women. To determine what's right for you, listen to your unique body rather than following the latest diet trend. The highest-quality sources are plant foods such as vegetables, fruits, legumes, and whole grains, which provide fiber, vitamins, minerals, and enzymes.

If you've considered a gluten-free approach, know that some women are genuinely sensitive to gluten or have celiac disease. Listen to your body, and if you suspect sensitivity, consider eliminating gluten for several weeks before reintroducing it to observe how you feel.

Many women in midlife discover that their carbohydrate tolerance changes. The bread that once caused no issues might now trigger bloating or fatigue. This isn't your body betraying you; it's offering you information about what serves you now, in this season of your life.

Fat: Your Essential Ally

Fat is not the enemy many women have been conditioned to fear.I t's an essential component of a nourishing diet, particularly during midlife when hormonal balance becomes increasingly important. Fats are vital building blocks for hormones, cell walls, brain tissue, and hundreds of chemicals that influence your physiology. They protect your internal organs, regulate body temperature and blood sugar, and provide insulation for your nerves.

Essential fatty acids are crucial for your nervous system, supplying energy and facilitating absorption of fat-soluble vitamins A, D, E, and K. When you restrict fat by using fat-free dressings to save calories, your beautiful salad becomes a nutritional wasteland.

Fat gives you a sense of fullness and satisfaction. It sustains you as it takes the longest to digest, creating warmth, nourishment, and pleasure. Opening yourself to pleasure without guilt is the ultimate gift of a healthy relationship with food and your body.

The fear that dietary fat automatically becomes body fat is both irrational and inaccurate. The fat stored on your body depends on the type and quality of fat you consume, not simply the amount. High-quality fats contribute to vibrant health, while poor-quality fats promote inflammation and imbalance.

Healthy fats include olive oil, sesame oil, coconut oil, avocados, wild fish, pasture-raised eggs, raw nuts, and seeds. When essential fatty acids are deficient, you might experience poor digestion, fatigue, dry skin and hair, joint pain, and decreased libido. Examples of poor quality fats are trans fats: artificial trans fats found in processed baked goods, margarine, and fast foods. They are linked to increased heart disease risk; hydrogenated oils: oils that have been chemically processed to be solid at room temperature, often containing trans fats; reused cooking oils: oils that have been repeatedly heated and used for frying can break down, forming harmful oxidation products; partially hydrogenated oils are used in some processed foods, these contain trans fats and should be avoided for better health. There is mixed research regarding saturated fats which are found in fatty cuts of red meat, lard, butter, there are those that tout the benefits of such and those that believe these fats can contribute to cardiovascular issues if consumed in large amounts. This is where you get to decide.

Marjorie, a fifty-five-year-old woman who came to me after decades of low-fat dieting, transformed her persistent dry skin, thinning hair, and frequent headaches by embracing healthy fats.

"I was literally starving my brain," she realized. "Adding avocados, olive oil, and nuts to my meals has changed everything. My skin glows, my thinking is clearer, and I finally feel satisfied after eating."

The Sacred Balance: Fat, Fiber, and Protein

To balance blood sugar, provide satiety, and maintain steady energy throughout your day, include a mix of fat, fiber, and protein in meals and snacks. This trio helps slow digestion, leading to more even glucose absorption, which keeps blood sugar balanced and helps you feel satisfied longer. This balance eliminates the energy highs and lows that can send you searching for quick fixes, perpetuating unhealthy cycles and feelings of anxiety.

The ideal mix varies for each woman. There's no secret formula; experiment with different combinations and tune into how your unique body responds.

Picture your plate as a canvas for this sacred balance. Perhaps a quarter holds protein—wild salmon, lentils, or pasture-raised eggs. Half your plate brims with colorful vegetables and fruits, fiber-rich and life-giving. The remaining quarter might include whole grains or starchy vegetables, like sweet potatoes or winter squash. Scattered throughout are the healthy fats such as olive oil drizzled over vegetables, avocado alongside your protein, and a sprinkle of seeds adding texture and nourishment.

This isn't a prescription but an invitation—an opportunity to play with proportions and discover what combination creates the most stable energy, clearest thinking, and deepest satisfaction for your unique body.

Fiber: Your Digestive Ally

Fiber from whole grains, nuts, seeds, legumes, vegetables, and fruits (rather than processed foods with added fiber) is essential for gut health, especially during midlife when digestive patterns often change. Fiber makes elimination easier, speeds transit time, dilutes toxins, removes harmful bacteria, and feeds beneficial bacteria that produce vital nutrients.

If you're increasing fiber intake, proceed gently and listen to your body's feedback. Start with less and work your way up to what feels right for you if digestion is uncomfortable. As a favorite mentor of mine has taught, "Start low and go slow."

Many women notice digestive changes during perimenopause and menopause, what once moved smoothly might now feel sluggish or unpredictable. Honoring these shifts by gradually increasing fiber can bring remarkable relief and restore digestive harmony.

Water: The Essence of Life

We can survive for weeks without food but only days without water. Your body is approximately seventy-five percent water, and you must continually replenish what's lost through activity and daily functioning.

Consider the water content of your food choices. Fruits and vegetables are hydrating, while breads and cereals are not. Herbal tea, soup, and some juices contribute to hydration, while caffeinated beverages can actually dehydrate. Insufficient water often manifests as low energy and false hunger signals.

A general guideline is consuming half your body weight in ounces daily. For a one-hundred and fifty -pound woman, aim for about seventy-five ounces, increasing with exercise or hot weather.

During midlife, proper hydration becomes even more crucial. Hot flashes and night sweats can deplete fluid levels rapidly. Adequate hydration supports joint health, cognitive function, skin elasticity, and kidney function—all of which may require extra attention during this season of life.

Consider creating beautiful rituals around hydration such as a special glass that brings you joy, infusing water with cucumber and mint, or beginning your day with warm lemon water as a gentle awakening for your digestive system. These simple practices make hydration fun instead of a chore.

The Energetics of Food: Beyond Nutrition

Food nourishes not only through nutrition but also through the experience and energy it creates. Each food carries its unique energetic imprint that you absorb alongside nutrients.

Steven Gagné explains in *The Energetics of Food* [1] that foods have distinct characteristics based on where they come from and how they grow. Green plants reach toward the sun, absorbing chlorophyll that oxygenates your blood and lifts your spirits. Squash grows close to the ground, offering mood-balancing properties. Root vegetables grow downward, providing grounding energy when you feel scattered.

This ancient wisdom offers another layer of understanding for your midlife nourishment. When you feel ungrounded or anxious—common during hormonal transitions—root vegetables like sweet potatoes, carrots, and beets might offer particular comfort. When your energy feels stagnant, leafy greens reaching skyward can help lift your spirits.

This perspective invites you to consider not just the chemical composition of your food but also its living energy—how it grew, where it came from, the hands that tended it, and the soil that

---

1. Gagné, Steven. The Energetics of Food: Encounters with Your Most Intimate Relationship. Spiral Sciences, 2006.

nourished it. This awareness transforms eating from mechanical fueling to sacred connection.

The Food-Mood Connection: Understanding Amino Acids and Neurotransmitters

The food-mood connection is profound. Some meals leave you feeling sluggish, while others elevate your energy and spirits. Brain chemistry influences mood through neurotransmitters like serotonin, which create relaxation, and dopamine and norepinephrine, which stimulate alertness.

Carbohydrate-rich foods release serotonin, creating relaxation (which explains why most binge episodes involve carbohydrates), but excessive amounts can cause drowsiness. Protein-rich meals release dopamine and norepinephrine, promoting alertness and focus, but too much can create tension. The gut actually sends more messages to the brain than the brain sends to the gut. Yes, your digestive system is truly your "second brain."

What many women don't realize is that food cravings and obsessions are often linked to brain chemistry imbalances. These imbalances involve specific chemical messengers called neurotransmitters that send impulses throughout your central nervous system, profoundly impacting your mental health, emotional state, and physiological functions.

The protein you eat provides amino acids—the essential building blocks for creating these neurotransmitters. When you're deficient in certain neurotransmitters, cravings and behaviors emerge as your body's way of self-medicating: [2]

- Low GABA or **Gamma-Aminobutyric Acid**levels may drive you to seek sugar to relieve anxiety and stress, creating temporary calm when you're worried or fearful.

- Low serotonin (sixty-five percent of which is produced in your gut) often triggers afternoon and evening cravings for sugar and carbohydrates, while also contributing to obsessive thoughts, excessive self-criticism, feelings of low self-worth, and digestive issues.

- Low catecholamines can make you crave sugar for energy, while low endorphins may lead you to eat for comfort and reward.

- Low glutamine appears as low blood sugar symptoms, causing cravings for sugar, starch, or even alcohol throughout the day, leaving you irritable, shaky, and headachy (hangry), with eating temporarily relieving fa-

---

2. Scott, Trudy. *The Antianxiety Food Solution: How the Foods You Eat Can Help You Calm Your Anxious Mind, Improve Your Mood, and End Cravings*. New Harbinger Publications, 2011.

tigue.

By addressing these underlying imbalances, you can help diminish and eventually eliminate cravings, along with the mood disorders related to neurotransmitter deficiencies. This approach breaks the vicious cycle of anxiety: eating→ temporary relief→ more anxiety.

If you choose to explore amino acid supplements to correct neurotransmitter deficiencies, work with a trained practitioner who can guide you to where you may be deficient, help you target and introduce them appropriately, and navigate away from potentially harmful interactions.

Your reaction to food is uniquely yours. Only you can determine the right balance of proteins, carbohydrates, and healthy fats for your optimal well-being.

Practice tracking your food and mood without judgment or obsession; it's simply a tool for gathering information about your body's wisdom as it responds to the foods you are choosing to eat.

Nurturing Through Life's Seasons

In midlife, our nutritional needs evolve with our changing hormones. The fluctuations of perimenopause and the stability of postmenopause both call for different approaches to nourishment.

During perimenopause, when hormones may swing dramatically, focusing on blood sugar stability becomes paramount. Regular meals containing that sacred balance of protein, healthy fat, and fiber can help minimize hot flashes, mood swings, and energy fluctuations.

Certain foods may support your body's production of estrogen during this transition:

- Flaxseeds contain lignans that can weakly mimic estrogen

- Fermented soy in forms like tempeh or miso provides phytoestrogens

- Cruciferous vegetables help with healthy estrogen metabolism

After menopause, bone health becomes an increasing priority. Foods rich in calcium, magnesium, vitamin D, and vitamin K support skeletal strength:

- Dark leafy greens provide calcium in a highly absorbable form

- Nuts and seeds offer magnesium that works with calcium for bone health

- Fatty fish supplies vitamin D for calcium absorption

- Fermented foods like sauerkraut contain vitamin K2 for proper calcium utilization

Again, these are not prescriptions but possibilities, and each woman's body responds differently to these transitions. Your work is discovering what serves your unique biochemistry as you move through these threshold moments.

From Control to Freedom: Beyond Willpower

As you move toward food freedom, incorporating these principles into your daily life, you'll discover a newfound energy that makes restrictive eating seem nonsensical by comparison.

Choice allows for confidence, and confidence inspires empowerment. Willpower, by contrast, is disempowering. As you begin this conversation with your body, approach it with curiosity, kindness, and compassion.

The journey to food freedom isn't linear.There will be days when old patterns resurface, when stress triggers familiar responses, when you find yourself returning to control rather than trust. In these moments, offer yourself the same compassion you would offer a dear friend. Each meal and each day offer a new opportunity to choose differently, to listen more deeply, and to trust more fully.

Remember that your body holds wisdom accumulated through decades of living. It knows more about what you need than any diet book, wellness influencer, or food trend. It takes a lifetime to learn to hear and honor its signals, deeply meaningful work that becomes increasingly rewarding as you become fluent in your body's unique language.

Your Invitation

I invite you to keep a gentle food/mood journal. Note what you eat, how you eat, and how you feel afterward, including any physical symptoms or emotional responses. Make this practice a mind/body/spirit exercise, releasing obsessive and judgmental thoughts.

As you write, notice patterns with curiosity rather than judgment and criticism. Perhaps you'll discover that certain foods leave you feeling energized while others create fatigue. You might realize that eating while distracted leads to digestive discomfort, or that meals enjoyed in company bring not just social connection but better digestion.

Consider these reflective questions as you journal:

- How do I feel physically after eating this meal?

- What emotions arise during and after eating?

- Do I feel satisfied, or am I still searching for something?

- What beliefs or thoughts accompanied this meal?

- How does my energy shift throughout the day in relation to what and when I eat?

Reflect on what nutritional beliefs you hold most strongly, and how might they evolve as you enter this new relationship with food? I've included a sample food logging journal in the resource section.

**Remember, my friend, your midlife metamor-
phosis isn't about restriction—it's about expansion into a more intuitive, peaceful relationship
with nourishment. You're not learning to control food; you're learning to trust yourself. This
journey to food freedom isn't just about what's
on your plate, it's about reclaiming your power,
pleasure, and peace with every mindful bite.**

In this luminous middle of life, you have earned the wisdom to
listen to your body with reverence. You have weathered enough
seasons to know that freedom comes not from rigid rules but
from flexible, compassionate attention to your changing needs.
You have lived long enough to understand that nourishment extends beyond calories and macronutrients to encompass pleasure,
connection, and celebration.

Now is the time to claim the freedom that comes from deep
alignment with your body's wisdom—to eat not from fear, but
from love; not from deprivation, but from abundance; not from
punishment, but from profound respect for the magnificent vessel
that carries you through this precious life.

Chapter Summary

In this liberating chapter, I invite you to release the rigid rules and restrictive eating patterns that have kept you trapped in a war with food. I explain how true nourishment honors our bio-individuality by recognizing that there is no single "right" diet for every woman, and introduces the essential macronutrients our bodies need, especially during midlife transitions.

The chapter explores the energetics of food, the profound food-mood connection through neurotransmitters, and how our nutritional needs evolve with hormonal changes. You learned that food freedom isn't about eating whatever we want without consideration for how it affects us, but rather making choices fueled by a desire to feel our best. This journey isn't about restriction but expansion into a more intuitive, peaceful relationship with nourishment—not learning to control food, but learning to trust ourselves.

Personal Reflection Exercises

Exercise 1: Releasing Nutritional Belief Systems

This exercise helps you identify and examine the food rules that may be limiting your relationship with nourishment.

1. **Identifying Your Food Rules:**

   ○ Create a list of all the food rules you currently follow or have followed in the past

   ○ Include rules from formal diets, family messages, cultural beliefs, and self-imposed restrictions

   ○ Be specific, noting exactly what each rule dictates (e.g ., "I must never eat after 7 p.m.," "Carbs are bad." "Fat makes you fat.")

2. **Exploring Rule Origins:**

   ○ For each rule, note when and where you first learned it

   ○ Identify whether it came from a diet program, a family member, media, a health professional, etc.

   ○ Consider what was happening in your life when you adopted this rule

3. **Assessing Impact:**

- For each rule, reflect honestly: Has following this rule consistently led to greater physical well-being? Mental peace? Emotional balance?

- Has the rule created stress, anxiety, or a sense of failure?

- Has it enhanced or diminished your enjoyment of food and eating?

4. **Transformation:**

- Choose one rule that feels particularly restrictive or has created suffering

- Create a new, more compassionate approach that honors both your body's needs and your life's realities

- Example: "I can't eat carbs" might become "I choose carbs that provide sustained energy and notice how different sources affect my unique body."

Exercise 2: Bio-Individuality Exploration

This exercise helps you discover what truly nourishes your unique body.

1. **Food Response Journal:** For one week, create a simple tracking system with these categories:

- Foods eaten

- Time of day

- Hunger level before eating (1-5 scale)

- Physical sensations after eating (30 minutes and 2 hours later)

- Energy levels after eating

- Mood changes

- Digestive responses

- Sleep quality (if applicable)

2. **Pattern Recognition:** After a week, review your journal and highlight patterns:

   - Which foods consistently provide sustained energy?

   - Which foods lead to energy crashes?

   - Which meals leave you feeling satisfied longest?

   - Which foods seem to trigger digestive discomfort?

   - How does the timing of meals affect your energy and sleep?

1. **Creating Your Bio-Individual Nourishment Map:**
   Based on these patterns, create a personalized nourishment map that includes:

   - Foods that consistently support your energy and well-being

   - Eating patterns that work best for your body's rhythm

   - Combinations of protein, fat, and carbohydrates that provide optimal satisfaction

   - Foods that your unique body may be sensitive to

   - How your needs might shift with hormonal cycles, seasons, or stress levels

Remember, this map isn't a rigid diet plan but a living document that evolves as you continue to listen to your body's wisdom.

Exercise 3: The Sacred Balance Plate Practice

This exercise helps you experiment with the sacred balance of protein, fat, fiber, and carbohydrates that I describe.

1. **Gather a set of small plates or bowls (or draw circles on paper)**

2. **Create different arrangements representing possible meal compositions:**

- Traditional balanced plate: ¼ protein, ¼ starchy carbohydrates, ½ non-starchy vegetables

- Higher protein approach: ⅓ protein, ⅓ healthy fats, ⅓ vegetables

- Plant-based approach: ½ vegetables, ¼ plant protein, ¼ whole grains with healthy fats incorporated

3. **Meal Planning Experiment:** Plan 3-6 meals using these different templates, making sure each includes:

- Quality protein sources

- Healthy fats

- Fiber-rich foods

- Complex carbohydrates (as appropriate for your body)

4. **Implementation and Reflection:**

- Try these different meal compositions over the course of a week

- After each meal, note:

  - How satisfied you feel

  - How stable your energy remains

- How your digestion responds

- How your mood is affected

  ○ At the end of the experiment, reflect on which balance
    seems to work best for your unique body

Exercise 4: Neurotransmitter Awareness

This exercise helps you explore potential connections between
your food cravings, mood patterns, and possible neurotransmitter
imbalances.

Create a personal assessment chart with these categories:

Serotonin Indicators:

- Do you experience afternoon/evening carbohydrate cravings?

- Do you struggle with obsessive thoughts or excessive
  self-criticism?

- Do you have trouble falling or staying asleep?

- Do you experience digestive issues?

- Do you feel anxious, worried, or fearful without clear
  cause?

GABA Indicators:

- Do you feel anxious, tense, or stressed much of the time?

- Do you crave sugar when feeling anxious?

- Do you have trouble relaxing or turning off your mind?

- Do you experience muscle tension or pain?

- Do you use food to calm yourself?

Catecholamines Indicators:

- Do you struggle with focus and concentration?

- Do you feel fatigued even after adequate sleep?

- Do you crave sugar for energy?

- Do you feel "flat" or uninspired?

- Do you rely on caffeine to feel alert?

Endorphin Indicators:

- Are you highly sensitive to emotional or physical pain?

- Do you eat for comfort and reward?

- Do you have trouble stopping once you start eating certain foods?

- Do you use food to soothe yourself when upset?

- Does eating provide temporary emotional relief?

For each category, note how many indicators resonate with your experience. If multiple indicators in any category ring true, this might suggest an area to explore further with a qualified health practitioner.

Journal Prompts

1. **Beyond the Battle:** I invite you to "end the exhausting war with food that has consumed precious energy better spent on living your most vibrant life." Reflect on how much mental and emotional energy your relationship with food currently consumes. What might become possible in your life if you could redirect this energy?

2. **Midlife Body Wisdom:** The chapter describes how during midlife, "The body that could once seemingly process anything without complaint now speaks to us with more urgency and clarity." What messages has your body been sending you about nourishment that you may have been ignoring? How might these messages be invitations to deeper listening rather than signs of betrayal?

3. **Quality vs. Quantity:** I challenge the idea that dietary fat automatically becomes body fat, noting that, "The fat stored on your body depends on the type and quality of fat you consume, not simply the amount." How might shifting your focus from quantity (calories, portions, weights) to quality (nutrient density, freshness,

how food is grown or raised) transform your relationship with eating?

4. **Food Energetics:** Consider the concept that foods carry unique energetic properties beyond their nutritional composition. Reflect on times when you've noticed how different foods affected not just your physical energy but your emotional or mental state. How might incorporating this awareness influence your food choices?

5. **Freedom vs. Indulgence:** "Where is the joy if what you're choosing leaves you feeling unwell? Can you reframe your beliefs about what truly satisfies?" Explore the difference between momentary pleasure that leads to physical discomfort and choices that provide both immediate enjoyment and lasting well-being. What does true food freedom look like for you?

Practice: The Sacred Meal Experiment

This week, create at least three sacred meals that incorporate not just nutritional wisdom but also mindfulness, pleasure, and connection.

Preparation:

1. **Select Your Meals:** Choose three meals during the week that can be unrushed and intentional

2. **Create Your Space:** Arrange your eating environment

to support presence (perhaps a cleared table, a candle, beautiful dishes)

3. **Plan Your Menu:** Design each meal to include the sacred balance of protein, fat, fiber, and carbohydrates that feels right for your body

4. **Gather Quality Ingredients:** Choose the highest quality foods available to you

The Sacred Meal Process:

1. **Before the Meal:**

   ○ Take three deep breaths to center yourself

   ○ Acknowledge the sources of your food with gratitude

   ○ Set an intention for how you wish to nourish yourself

2. **During the Meal:**

   ○ Eat without distractions (no screens, reading, or multitasking)

   ○ Notice the flavors, textures, and sensations

   ○ Pause midway through to check in with your hunger and satisfaction

   ○ Appreciate the balance of nutrients on your plate

3. **After the Meal:**

- Note how you feel physically, emotionally, and energetically

- Observe how long the satisfaction lasts

- Express gratitude for the nourishment received

Reflection: After completing all three sacred meals, journal about:

- Differences between these meals and your typical eating experience

- How the sacred balance affected your energy and satisfaction

- What you learned about your body's preferences and needs

- How you might incorporate elements of this practice into everyday eating

This experiment isn't about creating perfect meals but about bringing greater awareness, intention, and compassion to your relationship with nourishment.

Food & Mood Tracking Template

Create a simple but comprehensive tracking system to explore the connections between what you eat and how you feel:

Daily Page Format:

Morning Check-in:

- Sleep quality (1-5)

- Waking mood (1-5)

- Physical sensations

- Intentions for nourishment today

For Each Meal/Snack:

- Time:

- Foods eaten:

- Hunger level before (1-5):

- Fullness after (1-5):

- Eating environment (where, with whom, distractions):

- Physical sensations (30 min after):

- Energy level (1-5):

- Mood (1-5):

- Digestive response:

Evening Reflection:
- Overall energy today (1-5)

- Overall mood today (1-5)

- Food choices I felt good about:

- Challenging moments:

- What my body is asking for tomorrow:

Weekly Integration: After tracking for at least 5-7 days, look for patterns:
- Which meals provided the most sustained energy?

- Which foods seem connected to mood fluctuations?

- What eating patterns support your digestion?

- How does the timing of meals affect your sleep and energy?

- What have you learned about your unique needs?

Remember that this tracking isn't about judgment or creating new rigid rules, it's about curiosity and developing a deeper conversation with your body's wisdom.

Liberation Through Nutritional Self-Care

This practice helps translate nutritional knowledge into practical self-care that supports your midlife journey:

For each area of nutritional self-care, identify:

1. What you're currently doing that serves you well

2. One small, sustainable addition you could make

3. A compassionate approach to implementation

Hormonal Support:

- Current supportive practices:

- One addition to consider:

- Compassionate implementation:

Energy Stability:

- Current supportive practices:

- One addition to consider:

- Compassionate implementation:

Digestive Peace:

- Current supportive practices:

- One addition to consider:

- Compassionate implementation:

Mood Balance:
- Current supportive practices:

- One addition to consider:

- Compassionate implementation:

Hydration:
- Current supportive practices:

- One addition to consider:

- Compassionate implementation:

Example: Energy Stability:
- Current supportive practices: I already include protein at breakfast

- One addition to consider: Adding healthy fats to my afternoon snack

- Compassionate implementation: I'll keep avocados, nuts, and olive oil accessible so I can easily add these to my existing snacks when I remember. If I forget, I'll simply notice how I feel and use that information as feedback, not criticism.

Remember that liberation comes through gentle evolution, not radical restriction. Each small step toward honoring your body's needs is a step toward food freedom.

Looking Forward

As you continue your journey through *Midlife Metamorphosis*, notice how the nutritional wisdom in this chapter complements the mindfulness practices, hunger awareness, and nurturing movement you've explored in previous chapters. Each element supports the others, creating a foundation for true food freedom.

Remember that transformation isn't about perfection but about presence—being willing to listen to your body with compassion, respond with wisdom, and trust the process of becoming more attuned to your unique needs. Your midlife body isn't betraying you but inviting you into a deeper conversation about what truly nourishes you in this season of life.

"This journey to food freedom isn't just about what's on your plate, it's about reclaiming your power, pleasure, and peace with every mindful bite." - Mindy

The Hunger Beyond Food

Finding True Nourishment in Midlife

What are you truly hungry for in this season of your life?

Many of us in midlife have spent decades caring for others, building careers, and perhaps neglecting the quiet voice within. We've learned to survive, but not always to thrive. We've become experts at nourishing everyone but ourselves.

To be nourished is to be sustained with what is necessary for life, health, and growth; to be cherished, fostered, and kept alive; and to be strengthened, built up, and promoted. This definition extends far beyond the food on our plates.

In midlife, this truth becomes even more profound. We are nourished by so much more than what we eat—whether at a table, standing before the refrigerator, in our beds, or at our computers. To experience the completeness and satisfaction of a well-fed soul, we must attend to all areas of our lives that feed and sustain us.

Have you noticed that when your body, mind, and spirit are engaged in a creative project or fulfilling relationship, your reliance on food naturally decreases? Being passionately involved in meaningful work or relationships creates exhilaration that fuels us differently.

Conversely, when you're unsatisfied with your relationships, career, or other life dimensions, you may depend on food to cheer, soothe, or sedate you. When your life lacks balance, no amount of food can feed you where you truly need nourishment.

When Food Becomes a Substitute for Living

Let me tell you about Lisa, a woman in her mid-fifties who was referred by her doctor as she struggled with digestive issues, diabetes, chronic joint pain, and obesity.

Having endured early childhood traumas, Lisa learned to numb herself and avoid triggering emotions. She excelled academically and professionally, earning her place at a high-powered law firm, where she often worked twelve to fourteen hours a day, feeling overworked and overwhelmed as she oversaw a large team.

Most days Lisa skipped lunch, mindlessly grabbing almonds or cookies from the office snack room. She developed the habit of ordering dinner from her car on the way home, where she lived with her husband and two teenage daughters. Arriving home after the family had eaten and dispersed to various activities, Lisa finally felt she could breathe and enjoy some serenity.

It's important to note that when you're disconnected from your body, you don't pay attention to how your very wise body responds to the food you choose. Additionally, Lisa's comfort foods ignored the fact that she was gluten intolerant.

Lisa's need to self-soothe was perfectly valid, yet her desire to check out created consequences that only served to create additional issues. Not only was she worried about her health, but her relationships were suffering, and she had serious concerns about the behavior she was modeling for her daughters.

Can you see how her feelings and needs were showing up as wanting the food? As if the food was that emotional placeholder for the feelings that needed to be expressed.

Can you relate?

The temporary pleasure from highly refined, sugar-laden food creates a biological response that is powerful. It generates sensations of pleasure, reward, and relaxation. When this response subsides, the emotions return, you go back for more soothing, and the destructive cycle continues.

The desire is not for the food but for the distraction it creates and the avoidance of feelings believed to be intolerable.

In such instances, it's imperative to initiate a pause and ask, "What is going on? What am I really hungry for?"

A Path to Awareness

When Lisa learned to engage in the simple exercise introduced earlier—the PAUSE technique—she created space to discover what was really happening inside her:

P = Pause: Stop and take a full breath

A = Awareness: Notice what you're feeling physically and emotionally

U = Understand: Ask, "What do I need right now?"

S = Select: Choose a response that truly addresses this need

E = Evaluate: After responding, notice how you feel

This exercise created a huge "aha" moment for Lisa. She began to think differently about self-care and instituted changes in how she designed her life. Coaching helped her understand and honor her need to self-soothe, find safety within, and embrace where she felt secure today.

Now, on most days, Lisa's husband joins her for a planned dinner delivered from a local service. They even engage in meal prep together on weekends, including their daughters and talking honestly about root causes driving her relationship with food. Lisa is finding comfort in caring for herself and her hunger in ways that are neither self-sabotaging nor destructive.

As she started bringing lunch to work, she took time to stop and experience her food, honoring the physical hunger that deserves attention. With added probiotics unique to her physiology, gut-healing supplements, and menu options sufficient in appropriate protein, healthy fat, and fiber, her blood sugar has balanced, her mood has stabilized, and her anxiety has diminished. She feels lighter in her being, and as a result, her body is becoming lighter.

Healing Beyond Symptoms

I want you to know that healing is NOT simply about the end of symptoms. It's not about weight, nor is it about food groups. It's highly nuanced. It's about understanding your true self and discovering your uniqueness.

Compulsive behaviors and obsessive thoughts rob you of your ability to connect to the deepest part of yourself. True healing allows for acceptance—accepting your body size and shape rather than feeling diminished by it, accepting that eating is essential for life, and accepting the present moment so you can respond appropriately rather than numbing yourself.

Reframing your belief system and letting go of thoughts, feelings, and behaviors that, while once self-soothing, no longer serve you allows you to create the fully nourished life you desire and deserve.

The Foundation of All Relationships

The most fundamental relationship is the one you have with yourself.

This relationship affects all others—with family, friends, partners, and colleagues. Your struggles with weight and food have become an illustration of unavailability. For reasons unique to your journey, you've felt alone and outside, erected walls, and then felt even more isolated.

Whether your challenges stem from fear-based living, undigested trauma, or feelings of inadequacy, understand this: until you open up to receiving nourishment from yourself and your relationships, lasting freedom with food remains elusive.

Disordered eating and compulsive behaviors—whether restricting or overeating—cause isolation through shame. In that aloneness, self-destruction becomes easier as the voice urging indulgence grows louder than your true self, which ultimately craves human connection.

Being alone differs radically from isolating. Cultivating peaceful solitude provides a safe and sacred home you can continually return to, whereas isolating means building walls that perpetuate negative self-talk.

Clearing Space for Nourishment

Don't wait for a new season to clear what no longer serves you. Starting today examine your surroundings and identify what you're holding onto unnecessarily. Just as we release outdated clothing, we must release toxic relationships, limiting beliefs, and unrealistic expectations.

While doing so, clear your heart as well. Discard negative thoughts and detach from familiar but unhelpful narratives. Ask yourself whether these habits and beliefs serve any useful purpose. A clean, open heart welcomes all the goodness each day offers. Like rooms in your home, a cluttered heart and mind have no space for life's gifts and surprises.

Cherished memories remain forever in hearts and minds, but objects don't define us. Painful memories can teach meaningful lessons only when we clear space for healing. Releasing the past welcomes the energy of a healthy future.

The Power of Awareness

Throughout this book, I've emphasized awareness: awareness of blessings, of thoughts becoming beliefs, of what's true, of hunger and its origins, of who you are at the table, and of your body's wisdom.

While acknowledging that thoughts are merely thoughts, not facts, awareness lets you recognize your internal experience without being defined by it. This recognition leads to compassionate acceptance, which fosters hope and hope nurtures belief in manifesting your deepest desires.

I confidently state that if you've journeyed this far with me, you're aware of carrying significant burdens. This awareness marks the first step toward transformation. Without it, we remain stagnant; growth is impossible. Awareness brings clarity and direction, leading to the peaceful and joy-filled heart I wish for you.

What you might not realize is that you've arrived at this point, ready to claim your freedom, already whole. Perhaps after years of building protective layers, you've forgotten your core essence. Awareness reconnects you to this center, aligning you with life's wonder and nourishment.

Even when facing disappointment, grief, confusion, or personal challenges, we can transform our relationship to circumstances and positively influence our experience (what psychologists call post-traumatic growth).

This growth teaches boundary-setting, conscious choice-making, and integrity as we move forward without fear. Inspired awareness and compassionate acceptance allow transformation of habits that may no longer serve us. We freely release and relax into uncertainty with newfound faith.

Your Freedom Awaits

Renew your relationship with food now. A healthy relationship with food reflects a healthy relationship with life.

A healthy appetite for food and for life deserves honor as a fundamental act of self-love. Feed that hunger rather than fear it. Embrace a truly nourished and extraordinary journey through midlife and beyond. This is where healing happens.

For today and every day forward:

- Commit to consuming something positive daily. Find a teacher, mentor, book, blog, or community that inspires and uplifts you. Even a few words of daily inspiration matter—you literally become what you consume.

- List ways to reach out and strengthen connections with others, either mentally or in your journal.

The Beginning, Not The End

As this guide to your journey to food freedom concludes, it marks your beginning—the start of a joyful relationship with food, health, and spirit.

We've covered substantial territory, but remember: a healthy relationship with food builds on practicing gratitude for what you have while releasing stories that are no longer beneficial.

- You've explored the magnificent wisdom of questioning and experiencing feelings, even uncomfortable ones.

- You've embraced honoring physical hunger and appreciating your appetite as a life force rather than rejecting it.

- You've discovered the importance of slowing down, being

mindful, and recognizing body wisdom instead of wishing your body away.

- You understand the strong physiological connection between gut and brain, and you've embodied the profound wisdom that emerges in midlife.

- Finally, you understand that nourishment extends beyond food.

I won't deceive you by promising an obstacle-free path. For many of us, our food behaviors served meaningful purposes, keeping us in perceived safety.

You may have heard that your struggle with food isn't really about food, and perhaps you've heard without truly hearing. I confirm this statement to be absolutely true.

When we focus on soul-level hunger, we begin the journey to authentic nourishment. Unwanted eating habits eventually vanish once we no longer require food to control our emotions.

Begin returning home to your soul, where true nourishment resides, where you love and value yourself too much to inflict harm through hurtful thoughts or habits. Your true beauty, your radiance, emanates from within.

The midlife woman who nourishes herself with love and intention becomes the most powerful force in her life—and often, in the lives of many others. Your metamorphosis isn't just for you; it's a gift to everyone whose life you touch.

The bench awaits us both, whenever you need to rest.
To listen to life's music, breathe deeply, and be still.
The journey continues with its challenges and joys,
But remember—you need never walk alone.
Take my hand when you need support,
And know that your own hands now hold
The nourishment you've always sought.
  -Author Unknown

Chapter Summary

In this chapter, we explore the profound understanding that true nourishment extends far beyond what we eat. I invite you to recognize that many of your struggles with food stem from deeper hungers such as for connection, meaning, rest, joy, and self-acceptance. Through Lisa's story, we see how food can become a substitute for living fully when our lives lack balance or when we're disconnected from our deeper needs.

You also see how a client used the PAUSE technique that was introduced in earlier chapters. I emphasized that healing isn't simply about eliminating symptoms or achieving a certain body size but about accepting ourselves fully and creating space for authentic nourishment in all areas of life. The chapter concludes with a powerful reminder that our journey to food freedom is not an end but a beginning—an invitation to live with greater presence, joy, and self-compassion.

Personal Reflection Exercises

Exercise 1: Your Hunger Beyond Food

This exercise helps you identify areas of life where you may be seeking nourishment through food rather than addressing deeper needs:

1. **Create a "Hunger Inventory"** by reflecting on these questions:

   - When do you find yourself eating when not physically hungry?

   - What emotions typically precede these eating episodes?

   - What situations or environments trigger non-hungry eating?

   - What are you truly seeking in those moments? (Connection? Rest? Joy? Comfort? Safety? Recognition?)

   - What non-food experiences reliably satisfy each of these deeper hungers?

2. **Identify Your Nourishment Areas**
   Rate your satisfaction (1-10) in each of these areas of nourishment:

- Physical: Movement that brings joy, rest, touch, time in nature

- Emotional: Expressing feelings, receiving support, setting boundaries

- Intellectual: Learning, creativity, problem-solving, growth

- Social: Meaningful connection, belonging, community, intimacy

- Spiritual: Purpose, meaning, connection to something larger

- Vocational: Meaningful work, contribution, using your gifts

3. **Create Your Nourishment Plan**

For the 2-3 areas with the lowest satisfaction ratings:

- Identify one small action you could take this week to increase nourishment

- Consider what obstacles might arise and how you'll address them

- Set a specific time to incorporate this nourishment into your schedule

Exercise 2: Clearing Space for Nourishment

This exercise helps you identify and release what no longer serves you to create space for true nourishment:

1. **Physical Space Clearing**

   ○ Identify one small area in your home that feels cluttered or chaotic (a drawer, countertop, corner of a room)

   ○ Set a timer for 15-30 minutes to clear and organize this space

   ○ Notice how you feel before, during, and after this process

   ○ Consider: How might this physical clearing relate to your relationship with food?

2. **Mental Space Clearing**

   ○ List beliefs or thoughts about food, body, or self-worth that feel limiting or outdated

   ○ For each belief, ask: "Is this actually true? Where did I learn this? Does holding this belief serve my wellbeing now?"

   ○ Create an alternative thought that feels more aligned

with the person you're becoming

3. Relationship Space Clearing

- Reflect on your current relationships: Which ones feel nourishing? Which ones deplete you?

- Identify one boundary you could set to create more space for nourishment

- Consider one relationship you'd like to deepen or one new connection you'd like to cultivate

4. Time Space Clearing

- Review how you've spent your time over the past week

- Identify activities that felt depleting versus nourishing

- Choose one time-consuming activity that doesn't serve your wellbeing that you could reduce

- Identify one nourishing activity you could add with the time you free up

Exercise 3: Creating Your Nourishment Vision

This exercise helps you articulate and move toward a vision of a fully nourished life:

1. **Visioning Exercise**

   Close your eyes and imagine yourself one year from now, living in a way that feels deeply nourishing on all levels. Take your time to explore this vision:

   ○ How do you start your day?

   ○ How do you relate to food and your body?

   ○ What brings you joy?

   ○ How do you connect with others?

   ○ What gives your life meaning and purpose?

   ○ How do you care for yourself?

2. **Vision Articulation**

   Write a detailed description of this vision in present tense, as if you are already living it. Begin with: "I am nourished in body, mind, heart, and spirit. I..."

3. **Bridge Building**

   Identify the gap between your current reality and your vision:

   ○ What one aspect of this vision feels most compelling or important?

   ○ What is one small step you could take this week toward

this aspect?

- ○ What support might you need to sustain movement toward this vision?

- ○ What potential obstacles might arise, and how might you navigate them?

4. **Visual Representation**

Create a visual reminder of your nourishment vision:

- ○ This could be a collage, a drawing, a single word or phrase, or a collected object

- ○ Place this representation somewhere you'll see it daily

Journal Prompts

1. **Beyond Food Satisfaction:** You read "When your life lacks balance, no amount of food can feed you where you truly need nourishment." Reflect on a time when you tried to meet a non-food need with food. What were you truly hungry for? How might you have addressed that deeper hunger more directly?

2. **The Safety of Disconnection:** The chapter discusses how disconnection from our bodies and emotions can feel like safety. In what ways have you used food or body focus to avoid feeling difficult emotions? What might be-

come possible if you allowed yourself to feel these emotions with compassion?

3. **Midlife Wisdom:** Mindy suggests that midlife offers unique wisdom and opportunity for transformation. What wisdom have you gained through your life journey that you can now apply to your relationship with food and body? What aspects of yourself are ready to emerge in this phase of life?

4. **True Self-Care:** Our culture often conflates self-care with indulgence or numbing. Reflect on the difference between true nourishment and temporary comfort. What forms of genuine self-care leave you feeling truly replenished rather than needing more?

5. **The Foundation Relationship:** "The most fundamental relationship is the one you have with yourself.". How would you describe your relationship with yourself right now? If you treated yourself with the same care, respect, and attention you offer to someone you deeply love, what might change?

Practice: The Daily Nourishment Ritual

This practice helps you incorporate mindful awareness of your needs beyond food into daily life:

Morning Check-In (3-5 minutes)

1. **Body Connection:** Place one hand on your heart and one on your belly. Take three deep breaths.

2. **Physical Nourishment Awareness:**

   - Notice any physical sensations in your body

   - Consider: "What does my body need today?"

   - Identify one way you'll honor your body's needs today

3. **Emotional Nourishment Awareness:**

   - Notice any emotions present without judgment

   - Consider: "What does my heart need today?"

   - Identify one way you'll honor your emotional needs

4. **Purpose Nourishment:**

   - Consider: "What matters most to me today?"

   - Identify one small action aligned with your values

Mid-Day Check-In (2-3 minutes)

1. **Quick Body Scan:** Notice any physical sensations, particularly hunger/fullness cues

2. **Emotional Weather Check:** Name any emotions present without judgment

3. **Mindful Choice:** Ask, "What would truly nourish me right now?"

Evening Reflection (5 minutes)

1. **Gratitude:** Note one way you nourished yourself well today

2. **Learning:** Reflect on one challenging moment and what it might be teaching you

3. **Intention:** Set one simple intention for nourishment tomorrow

Practice this ritual daily for at least one week, noticing how your awareness of your needs shifts over time.

The Circle of Nourishment Practice

This reflective exercise helps you identify and strengthen your sources of nourishment beyond food:

1. **Draw a large circle on a blank page.**

2. **Within this circle, draw six sections labeled**

- Physical Nourishment

- Emotional Nourishment

- Mental/Intellectual Nourishment

- Social Nourishment

- Spiritual Nourishment

- Creative Nourishment

3. **For each section:**

- Write 1-2 activities that reliably nourish you in this area

- Note when you last engaged in each activity

- Rate your current satisfaction in this area (1-10)

- Identify one small way to increase nourishment in this area

4. **Integration Questions:**

- Which areas of nourishment feel most abundant right now?

- Which areas feel most depleted?

- What patterns do you notice between areas of depletion and your relationship with food?

○ What small shift in one area might create the most positive impact?

5. **Action Plan:**

○ Choose one area to focus on this week

○ Schedule a specific time for one nourishing activity in this area

○ After the activity, note how it affected your overall sense of nourishment and your relationship with food

This practice helps you see the interconnection between different forms of nourishment and creates awareness of how non-food nourishment impacts your relationship with eating.

Looking Forward

As you complete this workbook journey through *Midlife Metamorphosis*, remember that true transformation is not a destination but an ongoing process of awakening to your wisdom and worth. The practices, reflections, and insights you've gathered are not meant to be perfect performances but rather gentle invitations to live with greater awareness and compassion.

Your journey to food freedom is ultimately a journey home to yourself—to the wisdom that has always lived within you, perhaps waiting for this very moment to be fully expressed. As you read, "Your true beauty, your radiance, emanates from within. The midlife woman who nourishes herself with love and intention becomes the most powerful force in her own life—and often, in the lives of many others."

May you continue to discover all the ways you hunger for a rich and meaningful life, and may you nourish yourself fully as you move forward on this sacred path of transformation.

"When we focus on soul-level hunger, we begin the journey to authentic nourishment. Unwanted eating habits effortlessly vanish once we no longer require food to control our emotions." - Mindy

What's Next For You?

I f you've gotten to this page, I invite you to take a moment to acknowledge how far you've come. The journey to transform your relationship with food and your body is deeply personal, and by reaching this point, you've already shown tremendous courage and commitment to your well-being. The tools and practices you've explored throughout these pages have laid a foundation, but like any meaningful journey, this is not the end but rather a beautiful beginning.

Continuing Your Transformation

The path forward is uniquely yours. Some women find that having learned these tools, they're ready to continue practicing independently. Others discover that additional support, guidance, and community can profoundly accelerate their healing and growth. Wherever you are on this spectrum is perfectly valid.

As you consider next steps, I invite you to tune into what your body and heart are telling you. What kind of support would feel nourishing right now? What would help you integrate these practices more deeply into your life?

The Power of One-on-One Coaching

Individual coaching creates a sacred space where your specific challenges, patterns, and goals receive undivided attention. Our work together is tailored exclusively to your needs, allowing us to dive deeper than any book possibly could.

Melissa, one of my clients shared, "Working with Mindy transformed how I approach not just food, but my entire relationship with myself. The personalized guidance helped me navigate challenges I couldn't solve on my own for years. I finally feel at peace with my body."

In our one-on-one sessions, we:

- Create customized strategies that honor your body's wisdom. We'll ditch diet rules and build sustainable practices that support your energy, emotions, and real life.

- Break free from the cycles that have kept you stuck, including the shame, guilt, and all-r-othing thinking rooted in toxic diet culture.

- Celebrate your wins without attaching them to weight or willpower.

- We build a compassionate toolkit for navigating triggers, setbacks,and the emotional layers of your relationship with food and your body.

- Adjust your path in real time. As your needs shift, so will your practices, which grow with you.

This option is ideal if you're seeking personalized accountability, deeper emotional healing work, or if you're navigating complex health considerations alongside your food relationship journey.

The Magic of Community: Group Programs

There's something extraordinarily powerful about healing in a community. My group program, *The Fully Nourished Circle*, brings together women walking similar paths, creating a space of shared understanding, mutual support, and collective wisdom.

Jen, who participated in an earlier group program said, "I was hesitant about group work, worried my issues were too personal. But hearing other women voice the very thoughts I'd been ashamed of was incredibly freeing. We laughed, sometimes cried, and all grew stronger together."

In our group programs, you'll experience:

- The comfort of knowing you're not alone in your struggles with food, body image, or worthiness. You'll be held in a community that gets it, without judgement.

- Witness others reclaim their power by watching real women unlearn harmful narratives and choose compassion over control.

- Gain motivation that comes from shared commitment by showing up together with honesty, courage, and care.

- The collective wisdom that only a community can offer-as we share our lived experiences, create new truths, disrupt toxic norms, and build a more liberated path.

Group programs provide many benefits similar to individual coaching but at a more affordable cost, allowing more women to access this transformative work. They're particularly well-suited if you thrive in community settings and find strength in shared experience.

Your Invitation to Transform

Whether you choose to continue this journey independently, join our supportive community, or work with me one-on-one, I honor your path. There is no single right way forward, only what feels authentic and supportive for you right now.

If you're feeling called to explore coaching options, I invite you to:

Schedule a complimentary connection call: https://p.bttr.to/3 6nzVUu.

This conversation helps you discover if we're the right fit for each other and which path might serve you best.

Enjoy this collection of recipes: https://the-freedom-promise. kit.com/recipes.

Subscribe to my newsletter for ongoing support, inspiration, and first access to new programs: https://thefreedompromise.com/newsletter.

Remember that seeking support isn't a sign of weakness—it's a profound act of self-care. Just as you wouldn't hesitate to work with a guide when exploring new terrain, having guidance on this intimate journey of healing your relationship with food and body can make the path clearer, more joyful, and ultimately more transformative.

Wherever your path leads next, know that I'm honored to have shared this part of your journey through these pages. You carry within you everything you need to heal, and I'm here whenever you'd like additional support along the way.

The Midlife Metamorphosis Integration Practice

This final practice helps you integrate the wisdom from the entire book journey:

1. **Journey Review:** Briefly reflect on each chapter of your journey:

2. The path to radical acceptance

3. Finding your enough, feeling the love and facing your feelings

4. The mind-body-gut connection

5. Honoring your hunger

6. The mindful path

7. Embracing movement that nurtures

8. Nourishment as liberation

9. Finding true nourishment

10. **For each area, note:**

    - One key insight that resonated deeply

    - One practice you found most helpful

    - One shift you've noticed in yourself

11. **Integration Reflection:** Consider how these elements weave together in your life:

    - How has your understanding of nourishment expanded?

    - What old stories or patterns are you ready to release?

    - What new possibilities are emerging?

    - How has your relationship with food shifted?

○ How has your relationship with yourself evolved?

12. **Commitment Creation:** Create a simple, compassionate commitment to yourself that honors your continuing journey:

  ○ "I commit to nourishing myself by..."

  ○ "I choose to remember that..."

  ○ "When I struggle, I will..."

13. **Celebration:** Take a moment to acknowledge your courage in undertaking this journey:

  ○ What are you proud of?

  ○ What deserves celebration?

  ○ How will you honor this milestone?

Food for Thought

Group Questions for Book Clubs, Practitioners, and Support Groups

The Path to Radical Acceptance

C ommunity is where transformation takes place. Even though your transformation is extremely personal, sharing it with other women fosters a sacred environment where wisdom grows and healing speeds up. The purpose of these discussion questions is to encourage deep dialogue that goes beyond superficial sharing; they are invitations to delve into the delicate areas of your relationship with food, your body, and yourself with like-minded individuals.

These questions will help you uncover insights, celebrate victories, and create space for the messy, beautiful process of coming home to yourself, whether you're meeting with your book club, a support group, or just a trusted friend over tea. Keep in mind that this is a place for genuine answers, not flawless ones. Allow these discussions to serve as a gentle stimulant for the ongoing development of your midlife metamorphosis.

Group Discussion Questions

Introduction

1. Mindy shares that her relationship with dieting began in her teens. When did your own awareness of dieting or body size begin, and what factors do you think influenced this timing in your life?

2. The author describes her recovery from disordered eating as "a gradual clearing of the mist" rather than a specific moment of transformation. How does this description resonate with your own experience of change and healing?

3. Radical acceptance is described as "acknowledging reality exactly as it is, even when it's painful." What makes radical acceptance so challenging when it comes to our bodies and our relationship with food?

4. Mindy writes that her eating disorder "wasn't the problem, it had become [her] solution to deeper struggles." How might your own food behaviors be attempting to solve other problems in your life?

5. The introduction mentions how the diet industry profits from women's dissatisfaction with their bodies. How has diet culture specifically targeted women in midlife? What messages about aging and body changes have you internalized?

6. Mindy shares that "no feeling is more uncomfortable than the discomfort of avoiding it." What emotions have you been avoiding through your relationship with food?

7. The author found that becoming a grandmother helped crystallize what truly matters to her. What life experiences have shifted your perspective on the importance of body size or appearance?

8. Mindy mentions that "HOW, WHY, and WHEN we eat profoundly impacts WHAT we eat." How have you observed this connection in your own life?

Chapter 1: Laying the Foundation

1. Mindy describes midlife as offering "the perfect combination of earned wisdom and remaining years to apply it meaningfully." How has your perspective on aging shifted over time, and what wisdom do you now value that came through life experience?

2. The chapter introduces Debi's story and how her family

associations with food being equated with love, comfort, and connection influenced her relationship with eating. How were food, emotions, and care connected in your family of origin? How do you see those patterns showing up in your life today?

3. Mindy writes about the shift from willpower to willingness as essential for transformation. How has relying on willpower affected your relationship with food, and what might a more willing approach look like for you?

4. The chapter discusses how we often use food to numb uncomfortable emotions. What emotions do you find most challenging to feel fully, and how has food played a role in helping you avoid them?

5. Mindy suggests that "your relationship with food mirrors your unique relationship with yourself and your story." What insights about your relationship with yourself have you gained by reflecting on your relationship with food?

6. The chapter introduces the concept of ancestral wisdom and non-negotiables for health. Which of these foundations (diet, sleep, exercise, breath, excretion, emotions) feels most important for you to strengthen right now, and why?

7. Mindy describes how practicing gratitude can transform our perspective from not enough to abundance. How has

gratitude (or the lack of it) influenced your experience with food and body image?

8. The chapter ends with the powerful image of Mindy walking on the beach, fully present and at peace with herself. What would your own version of this "coming home to yourself" moment look like?

Chapter 2: Eating Disorders in Midlife

1. The chapter opens by challenging the myth that eating disorders primarily affect young women. How has this misconception affected awareness, treatment, and support for midlife eating disorders? What unique barriers might prevent midlife individuals from seeking help?

2. The chapter discusses how care-giving responsibilities—for children, aging parents, or both—can contribute to disordered eating in midlife. How has the "sandwich generation" experience affected your relationship with self-care and nourishment? What would more balanced caregiving look like?

3. Hormonal transitions during midlife create real physical and emotional changes. How has perimenopause or menopause affected your relationship with your body and food? What wisdom might these transitions offer if approached with curiosity rather than resistance?

4. The chapter notes that over 88% of middle-aged women express substantial body dissatisfaction. How does sharing this struggle with others affect your experience of it? What might become possible through collective healing rather than isolated suffering?

5. Mindy defines recovery as "regaining what was lost or taken" and notes that obsessive thoughts and behaviors rob us of connection to our deeper selves. What aspects of yourself have been diminished by food and body preoccupation? What would you like to reclaim?

6. Radical acceptance involves embracing reality without judgment or resistance. What areas of your life beyond food and body might benefit from this approach? What fears arise when you contemplate radical acceptance? What possibilities might it open?

Chapter 3: Find Your Enough, Face Your Feelings, Feel the Love

1. The chapter suggests that "choosing foods that support her well-being isn't an act of restriction but an expression of self-respect." How does this perspective differ from traditional diet mentality? Can you recall a time when you made a food choice from self-respect rather than restriction? How did it feel different?

2. Mindy states that "limiting beliefs that hold us back are rooted in fear." What fears underlie your own limiting beliefs about food and body? What might become possible if you could release these fears?

3. The chapter explores how self-criticism blocks self-love. What forms of self-criticism most commonly appear in your relationship with food and body? What would it look like to approach these areas with compassion instead?

Chapter 4: The Mind-Body-Gut Connection

1. The chapter states that "your relationship with food often mirrors your more profound relationship with yourself and your life experiences." How have you observed this connection in your own life? What insights about yourself have you gained by reflecting on your eating patterns?

2. Mindy explains how the stress response evolved as a survival adaptation and can become problematic in modern life. What aspects of modern living do you find most challenging to your nervous system? How do these challenges affect your relationship with food?

3. The chapter describes the second brain in our digestive system and its communication with our central nervous system. Have you experienced this gut-brain connection

in ways beyond digestion (intuition, emotional responses, etc.)? How might honoring this connection change your approach to eating?

4. For those navigating perimenopause or menopause: How has your relationship with food changed during this transition? What new body wisdom have you discovered that wasn't part of your experience in earlier decades?

5. Mindy mentions the "French Paradox" and how the state of our nervous system during eating may be as important as what we eat. What cultural or family eating practices have you observed that support relaxed, present eating? How might you incorporate elements of these practices into your own life?

6. The chapter explains how chronic stress creates hormonal cascades that affect weight management and digestion. How does understanding these biological mechanisms change how you think about your body's responses to stress? Does this knowledge shift how you view your past experiences with food and weight?

7. Discuss Mindy's statement that "worrying about weight often increases weight, while relaxing into nourishment allows your body to find its natural balance." What has been your experience with this paradox? What makes relaxing into nourishment challenging in our current cul-

ture?

8. The chapter emphasizes that the path forward isn't found through rigid control but through cultivating presence and physiological balance. How does this approach differ from other health or nutrition advice you've encountered? What feelings arise when you consider releasing control around food?

Chapter 5: The Mindful Path to Radical Acceptance

1. Mindy begins the chapter by sharing her experience of counting pasta pieces while missing connection with her family. What similar experiences have you had where focusing on controlling food prevented you from being fully present? How did these moments affect your relationships with yourself and others?

2. The chapter describes how neuroplasticity during midlife creates an opportunity for transformation. What changes have you noticed in how you think about your body or food as you've entered or moved through midlife? What old patterns seem to be loosening their grip?

3. Mindy states that "pleasure becomes the cornerstone of food freedom." How does this perspective differ from conventional approaches to nutrition and health? What fears or resistance might arise when considering pleasure

as central to your relationship with food?

4. The chapter emphasizes how eating without awareness affects digestion and nutrient absorption. What multi-tasking habits have become part of your eating routine? How might prioritizing single-tasking during meals benefit your physical and emotional wellbeing?

5. Mindy distinguishes between a compulsive eater and a food lover, noting that "eating WITH emotion rather than eating TO manage emotions is transformative." How do you experience the difference between these two approaches? When have you experienced true pleasure and presence with food?

6. The neuroscience of self-compassion suggests that self-criticism activates our threat response, while kindness creates safety for change. How have you experienced this dynamic in your approach to food and body? What self-compassionate practices might support your healing journey?

7. The chapter introduces the concept of radical acceptance, embracing reality completely without resistance. What aspects of your relationship with food and body feel most challenging to accept? What possibilities might open if you could fully embrace where you are right now?

8. Mindy shares that her transformation came when she "no

longer feared what food would do TO me and fully embraced what it could do FOR me." How might shifting from fear to nourishment change your daily experience with food? What specific foods or eating situations might be transformed through this perspective shift?

Chapter 6: Honoring Your Hunger

1. Mindy describes how hunger is "not merely a physical sensation but a powerful evolutionary mechanism." How has your relationship with hunger evolved throughout your life? What factors have influenced whether you trust or distrust your hunger signals?

2. The chapter distinguishes between physical hunger, emotional hunger, and toxic hunger. Which of these types do you find most challenging to recognize in yourself? What specific body sensations help you identify each type?

3. Mindy states that "cravings represent your body's sophisticated communication system." Share an experience where a craving turned out to be a message about something your body or spirit truly needed. How did you decipher this message?

4. The chapter suggests that many of us have lost our connection to hunger wisdom due to our current food environment. What aspects of modern food culture make

it particularly challenging to maintain this connection? What strategies have you found helpful in reconnecting with your body's signals despite these challenges?

5. Mindy describes how childhood messages about cleaning your plate or consuming food quickly affected our ability to recognize fullness signals. What messages about eating did you receive as a child? How do these continue to influence your eating patterns today?

6. The chapter proposes that "giving yourself unconditional permission to eat anything" is the first step toward a peaceful relationship with food. What feels frightening or liberating about this idea? What beliefs or fears arise when you consider this approach?

7. Mindy suggests that "your relationship with food reflects how you work, connect with others, and care for yourself." How does your approach to food mirror other aspects of your life? What insights about yourself have you gained by reflecting on this connection?

8. The chapter emphasizes the importance of learning to say both "yes" and "no" with confidence. Where else in your life might you need to practice more balanced boundaries? How might healing your relationship with food support this broader work?

Chapter 7: Embrace Movement That Nurtures

Movement Wisdom Circle (Group Practice)

This practice is designed for group settings, creating a safe space to share experiences and wisdom about nurturing movement:

Preparation:

- Arrange chairs in a circle

- Have a talking piece (a stone, feather, or other meaningful object)

- Establish group agreements: confidentiality, non-judgment, speaking from personal experience, and listening with compassion

Opening:

- The facilitator briefly introduces the concept of movement as celebration rather than punishment

- Participants take three collective breaths to center themselves in the present moment

Sharing Rounds:

1. Memory Round: Share a memory of a time when movement brought you joy. (Each person shares briefly while holding the talking piece)

2. Wisdom Round: What has your body taught you

through movement that you couldn't have learned any other way?

3. Challenge Round: What harmful messages about exercise or movement do you have, and how are you releasing them?

4. Vision Round: What would a truly nurturing relationship with movement look like in your life going forward?

Integration:

- After all rounds, participants reflect together on common themes and insights

- Each person shares one small step they'll take in the coming week to move with more compassion and joy

Closing:

- The group stands in a circle and each person offers one word that represents what they're taking from the experience

- A final collective breath completes the practice

This circle creates space for collective wisdom to emerge while honoring each person's unique experience with movement and embodiment.

Chapter 8: Nourishment as Liberation

1. Mindy begins the chapter with an invitation to "release the weight of food fears you've carried for far too long." What food fears have been most burdensome in your life? How have these fears affected your relationship with eating and your body?

2. The chapter introduces the concept of bio-individuality—"there is no single 'right' diet for every woman." How does this perspective differ from mainstream approaches to nutrition? What resistance or relief do you feel when considering that your body's needs might be fundamentally different from others'?

3. Mindy describes how many of us have been taught to fear carbohydrates and fats. How have these fears manifested in your own relationship with food? What might change if you approached these macronutrients as potential allies rather than enemies?

4. The chapter explains how protein, fat, and fiber work together to create stable energy and satisfaction. When have you experienced the benefits of this balanced approach? What challenges have you encountered in finding your own optimal balance?

5. Mindy notes that "during midlife, our relationship with

food often undergoes profound transformation." How has your body's response to different foods changed as you've moved through various life stages? How have you navigated these changes?

6. The chapter discusses the food-mood connection, explaining how neurotransmitter imbalances can drive specific food cravings and behaviors. How does understanding this biological basis affect how you think about willpower and self-control around food?

7. Mindy suggests that "each food carries its unique energetic imprint that you absorb alongside nutrients." How does considering food's energetic properties expand your understanding of nourishment beyond nutritional science? What foods feel most energetically aligned with your current needs?

8. The chapter concludes by emphasizing that the journey to food freedom isn't linear and requires compassion when old patterns resurface. Where in your relationship with food could you benefit from greater self-compassion? What would this compassion look and feel like in practice?

Chapter 9: The Hunger Beyond Food

1. Mindy opens the chapter by asking, "What are you tru-

ly hungry for in this season of your life?" What deeper hungers are you aware of beyond physical food? How might addressing these hungers directly impact your relationship with food?

2. The chapter describes how many of us in midlife "have spent decades caring for others, building careers, and perhaps neglecting the quiet voice within." How has this shown up in your life? What is that quiet voice within you asking for now?

3. Lisa's story illustrates how food can become a substitute for addressing deeper needs. What aspects of her story resonated with your own experience? What insights did her journey offer you?

4. Mindy writes that "healing is NOT simply about the end of symptoms. It's not about weight, nor is it about food groups." How does this perspective differ from conventional approaches to healing your relationship with food? What shifts when you focus on nourishment rather than restriction?

5. The chapter discusses how compulsive behaviors and obsessive thoughts disconnect us from our true selves. In what ways have food rules or body preoccupation created distance from your authentic self? What aspects of yourself have been waiting to be expressed?

6. Mindy suggests that clearing space in various areas of life creates room for true nourishment. What areas of your life feel cluttered or depleting? What might become possible if you created more space?

7. "When we focus on soul-level hunger, we begin the journey to authentic nourishment. Unwanted eating habits effortlessly vanish once we no longer require food to control our emotions." What has been your experience with addressing deeper needs and how it affects your relationship with food?

8. The chapter concludes by saying "The midlife woman who nourishes herself with love and intention becomes the most powerful force in her own life and often, in the lives of many others." How might your own healing journey impact those around you? How might your food freedom create ripples beyond your own life?

Resources

Recommendations for Further Reading

Jonathan Bailor, *The Calorie Myth*, Harper Collins, 2014

Byron Katie and Steven Mitchell, *Loving What Is*, New York, Three Rivers press, 2002

Thomas Moore, *The Dark Night of the Soul: A Guide to Finding Your Way Through Life's Ordeals*, USA,Gotham Books, Penguin Group, 2005

Mary O'Malley, *The Gift of Our Compulsions*, California, New World Library, 2004

Julia Ross, *The Mood Cure: The 4 Step Program to Re-balance Your Natural Sense of Well-Being*, New York, Penguin Group, 2002

Geneen Roth, *Women, Food and God*, New York, Scribner, 2010

Geneen Roth, *When Food Is Love*, New York, Plume, The Penguin Group, 1992

Don Miguel Ruiz with Janet Mills, *The Four Agreements*, Amber-Allen Publishing, 1997

Free Guide: The Benefits of Essential Oils

Mood and Behavior Management for Your Journey to Food Freedom

E ssential oils support healing on many levels. As each level is healed, we prepare for the next level. For the individual challenged by and perhaps struggling with disordered eating behaviors, we must look at healing not only the physical body but the mind and spirit as well.

So often, disordered eating behaviors evolve as a result of limiting beliefs and a loss of spiritual and social awareness and connection.

As the disordered behaviors take root, the toll on the physical body is enormous.

Essential oils assist in the healing process as they purify organs and body systems, raising the body's vibration. They assist in allowing us to look inward at the emotional and psychological realm. As we have awareness, we can be more open to acceptance and compassion, allowing us to let go of the beliefs, messages, and ultimately, behaviors that are no longer serving us well.

Strong recovery starts with taking the necessary steps on the journey to healing. Self-discovery, journaling, personal inventory, and responsibility will all make the path easier to negotiate. Let essential oils energize you to become the most brilliant version of yourself.

The Freedom Promise introduces you to seven steps for food freedom. I'd like to briefly walk you through each step and assign the oils that will be most beneficial. Visit https://thefreedo mpromise.com/guidefor more information.

Find Your Enough, Feel the Love, Face Your Feelings

In this step we examine how gratitude sets the tone for how we perceive our lives. When we start each day aware of and grateful for what we have, rather than longing for what we don't, we can operate on a higher energy plane. Feelings are rooted in thoughts and beliefs. Many of those thoughts and beliefs develop from messages that we hold on to that have no significant meaning for us anymore. When we can explore the origin, find compassion for the message, and accept how it once served us, we can disengage and let it go. Finding your enough means believing that where you are now is where you are meant to be. It means you have a safe and sacred home within yourself to always return to.

Recommended Oils: Parasympathetic (grounding and present), Liver Support (releasing toxic emotions and beliefs) Orange(abundance) Small Intestine Support (self-acceptance), Heart or Rose (love & trust), Energize or Lymph (zest for life), Peppermint(buoyant heart), Thyroid Support (finding your voice)

Rest and Digest

This step deals with the effects of and science of stress. While stress is and always will be a part of life as we know it, successful stress management is about how we react to it. There are two parts of our central nervous system – the sympathetic (fight or flight) and the parasympathetic (rest and digest). In flight or flight mode, we experience digestive shut down, lack of nutrient absorption, not to mention elevated blood pressure, elevated cortisol and insulin levels which can contribute to adrenal fatigue. When in a rest and digest mode, all systems are functioning optimally and we experience the healthy flow that allows us to assimilate nutrients, efficiently metabolize and live in a rhythm that will bring optimal emotional and physical health.

Recommended Oils: Liver Support (release and forgiveness), Calm (relaxation) Adrenal (relief), Hypothalamus (realignment),

Kidney Support or Spleen Support (releasing fear and calming the inner child), Bladder Support (release and relief from trauma).

Since so much of the stress we feel while engaging in disordered eating behaviors is induced by negative self talk and a poor sense of self, we address these issues here with specific oils, as well.

Recommended: Lemon(focus), Parasympathetic (mindfulness and stability), Uplift (self-love and optimism).

Eat When You're Hungry, Stop When You've had Enough

This step is about honoring your hunger, which is essentially an appetite for life! Here we learn to recognize and honor true physical hunger as opposed to emotional hunger, which has us craving instant gratification for something to fill a void or help us to check out from an uncomfortable situation or trigger. Recommended Oils: Parasympathetic and Hypothalamus (connect with body) Small Intestine Support or Large Intestine Support (inner beauty, body acceptance), Blood Sugar Balance or Pancreas (curbs cravings to numb the senses and check out).

Eat Mindfully

This step is important as it reminds us of the importance of being present. Mindfulness is about being aware of the here and now, without judgment. When we bring mindfulness to the table, we can be fully engaged in the experience of eating; aware of how our senses are called upon to smell, taste and connect with our bodies as they become satiated. Mindfulness at the table does not allow for distraction from TV, computer, magazines, or even the negative thoughts that occur when we question what we are eating. Mindfulness encourages us to relax into the state where we most efficiently digest, metabolize and find pleasure in our food choices.

Recommended oils: Focus (presence + commit to the goal), Hypothalamus (connect to your physicality and actual hunger), Parasympathetic (grounding and centering).

Do Something Every Day That Makes Your Body Feel Alive

This step is about moving in an effort to honor your body as opposed to engaging in punishing exercise designed to make your body go away. Our bodies want to move, be lovingly nurtured and nourished.

Recommended Oils: Grapefruit(honor the body), Lymph and Parasympathetic (connect with the body), Energize or Adrenal (motivation)

Only Eat Whole Foods, or As Often As You Can

This step is about nourishing our bodies and embracing the energetics of food. Eating unprocessed, fresh, organic and seasonal foods ensures that we are fueling our bodies in the best way possible. The steps up to this point set us up for optimal nutrient absorption. This step gives us the macro- and micro-nutrients necessary for ideal health and well-being. Recommended: Parasympathetic, Digest blend, Gallbladder, Pancreas (to help release digestive enzymes), Intestinal Mucosa,

Make Sure You Surround Yourself With What Truly Nourishes

This step has us looking at how we live our lives in relation to how nourished we are. This kind of nourishment is not found in the kitchen. It comes from our relationships, career choices, spirituality, and physical activity.

Recommended Oils: Parasympathetic, (community), Frankincense or Rose (emotional healing), Uplift (protects against negative energy), Liver Support (vitality and transition from destructive behaviors), Hypothalamus (sexual purity and balance), Thyroid Support (spiritual purpose and finding your voice), Rose (Divine love), Brain Boost (sacred devotion and light), Uplift (mood stabilizing and joy), Orange (inspires play, relaxation and authenticity)

As a result of these steps you may experience a transformation that has you move out of the darkness into the light created by the most brilliant version of yourself. For this we recommend Frankincense (truth) Brain Boost (Faith and Grace) and Adrenal (Renewal)

To order your oils, please use this link https://dv216.isrefer.co m/go/VBO/a1090/..

*The Freedom Promise receives a small commission on the sale of the oils.

Acknowledgements

This dream of writing a second book would never have become a reality without Jennifer Grace, my publisher and publicist. Meeting her and being captivated by her warmth, sincerity, and encouragement propelled me to take action and put words to these pages. And then there is Raven Petty, Jennifer's partner and my editor, who has coached me, supported my message, and motivated me to dig deep. Her wisdom and intuitive insight have been an extraordinary gift.

My growth during the twelve years since I wrote *The Freedom Promise* has been in large part due to the women who openly share their lives with me and allow me to accompany them on their private and sacred journeys. I cherish every one of them and extend my heartfelt gratitude for this privilege. Every day, they inspire me to strive to be the best version of myself. To all of you, I hope I have captured your transformation in a way that inspires you to stay on the path and encourages others to take that difficult first step.

I have the most wonderful community of friends, colleagues, and mentors who have seen me through my metamorphosis; you know who you are. Your love and friendship will continue to envelop me. Andrea Nakayama and our extraordinary community of FNLPs, you lift me up and inspire me with your brilliance. Jen Gottlieb and Chris Winfield welcomed me into their Mastermind family and encouraged me daily to grow, take action, and expand my presence on this blessed earth. Thank you, Jen, for allowing me to experience what you teach—that "discomfort is temporary but growth is permanent."

Megan, my assistant and project manager has been an integral part of everything I do. Without her, none of my back-office operations would be possible.

My medical team at Long Island Jewish Hospital are my angels. Dr. Nicole Lapinel, Jess, Theresa, Katie, Christina and Sasha: I can only hope you know how much your care and support mean to me.

The Cystic Fibrosis Foundation community: I can't imagine there is a more devoted and conscientious group of individuals, who give of themselves tirelessly, during these tumultuous times of funding cutbacks and uncertainty.

Erin and Kayla, our relationship means the world to me. Mom is always with us and I know, she is so very proud of your magnificence. I am grateful that you allowed me to share a part of her journey.

Nothing I do is without forethought for, inspiration from, and motivation to be the best I can be for my family. I am so incredibly blessed to be living this big, beautiful life that sometimes feels like I am living in a kaleidoscope. My daughters and stepsons, sons-in-law, daughters-in-law, and our extraordinary grandchildren continue to be an enormous source of joy. We are a beautifully blended family, and I feel so very fortunate to honor and uphold my place in our family. Ricki and Jonathan, Dani and Yale, Amy and Mark, Alisha and Lee, Sarah, Spencer, Jake, Lexi, Hannah, Zach, Mia, and Mason, I love you with all my being, to the depths of my very deep soul.

Eddie, your encouragement and constant reminders of what is possible keep me grounded and have allowed me to become the change I so wanted to see. I love you with all of me.

Mindy
Gorman-Plutzer

W hat happens when thirty years of nutritional knowledge meets the gentle understanding of a woman who has gone through her own transformation? You get Mindy Gorman-Plutzer, a remarkable role model for women seeking to transform their perspectives on food, their bodies, and themselves.

Mindy's journey didn't start in a classroom or clinic; it started in the mirror, where she saw her problems with food and body image. She was stuck in the tiring cycle of diet culture's promises and failures, just like so many other women. But instead of accepting the present as her fate, she chose a different path that would eventually show thousands of others the way.

Mindy is now a Certified Functional Nutrition and Lifestyle Practitioner, a Board Certified Integrative Health Coach, and a Certified Eating Psychology Coach. But her most important credential is still her lived experience as a woman who has gone through the fire of food fear and come out with a message of radical self-acceptance.

Mindy has been working on her unique method for over 30 years at her private practice in New York. It is a groundbreaking system that respects both the science of nutrition and the sacred wisdom of the female body. She skillfully combines functional nutrition, psychology, mind-body science, and body-centered practices to create a concept she refers to as "empathetic empowerment." This practice is a kind and compassionate way to deal with the physical and emotional problems that come up because of our complicated relationship with food.

Mindy says, "My philosophy is to help my clients make healthy lifestyle and food choices by connecting with the healthy wisdom of their bodies." This isn't another diet or quick fix; it's about finding yourself again.

Mindy lives on Long Island with her husband. She is an avid golfer, Pilates enthusiast, and looks forward to her daily Wordle challenge.

Work With Mindy Gorman-Plutzer

Mindy is also the author of *The Freedom Promise: 7 Steps To Stop Fearing What Food Will Do TO You and Start Embracing What It Can Do FOR You* (Balboa Press). She has taken decades of clinical experience and personal insight and turned them into a guide to food freedom. Her work has affected many more lives than just those in her practice. She has reached women through her appearances on Doctor Radio, Huffington Post Live, ABC news.com/podcast, and a number of other radio shows that are broadcast to a wide audience.

Mindy's voice has been on the pages of Mind Body Green and The Fifty Plus Life, where she was a trusted contributor. She has been a popular guest expert at highly praised wellness summits, where she has shared her knowledge with women all over the world who are ready to change not only their relationship with food but also how they take care of and value themselves.

Her blog, https://thefreedompromise.com/blog/, where she writes with her usual warmth and insight about everything having to do with the mind, body, and spirit, has become a safe place for women searching for real help on their healing journey. Mindy continues to spread her message that real health isn't about being perfect; it's about being at peace. She does this through many podcast appearances and speaking engagements.

But maybe the most powerful thing about Mindy's work is that she knows that midlife is a time when women can change in a big way. She knows that this stage of life needs a different kind of growth—one that honors the lessons you've learned, the fights you've fought, and the woman you're becoming.

When you work with Mindy, you're not just getting a health coach; you're getting a caring guide who knows that your relationship with food is closely linked to your journey to find yourself. She knows that healing doesn't come from being forced or limited; it comes from the gentle art of returning to your body's wisdom.

"Wouldn't it be great to know that you can change your relationship with food from one full of fear and confusion to one full of joy, love, and freedom?"

Mindy wants you to do more than just read about change; she wants you to live it. *Midlife Metamorphosis* gives you the tools you need to have a relationship with food and your body that is not only healthy but also good for your soul.

Your metamorphosis is coming. Mindy is here to help you get home.

You can find her on:

Instagram @thefreedompromise

Facebook www.facebook.com/thefreedompromise

LinkedIn @Mindy Gorman-Plutzer

Her podcast *SoulShift* is available on your favorite podcast platform, or find the video version on her YouTube channel, The Freedom Promise with Mindy Gorman-Plutzer.

Web: https://thefreedompromise.com

Email: mindy@thefreedompromise.com